T0160387

IT'S NOT ABOUT THE

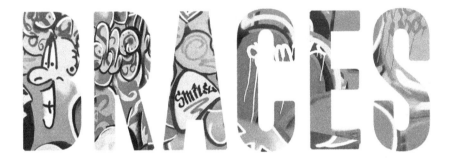

IT'S NOT ABOUT THE

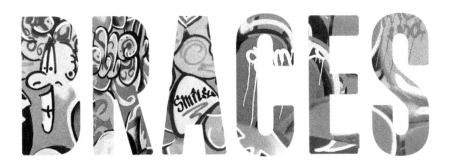

A GUIDE TO YOUR ORTHODONTIC QUESTIONS

W. CLARK ANDERSEN, DDS

Advantage®

Copyright © 2021 by W. Clark Andersen.

All rights reserved. No part of this book may be used or reproduced in any manner whatsoever without prior written consent of the author, except as provided by the United States of America copyright law.

Published by Advantage, Charleston, South Carolina.
Member of Advantage Media Group.

ADVANTAGE is a registered trademark, and the Advantage colophon is a trademark of Advantage Media Group, Inc.

Printed in the United States of America.

10 9 8 7 6 5 4 3 2 1

ISBN: 978-1-64225-200-2
LCCN: 2021906218

Book design by Wesley Strickland.

This publication is designed to provide accurate and authoritative information in regard to the subject matter covered. It is sold with the understanding that the publisher is not engaged in rendering legal, accounting, or other professional services. If legal advice or other expert assistance is required, the services of a competent professional person should be sought.

Advantage Media Group is proud to be a part of the Tree Neutral® program. Tree Neutral offsets the number of trees consumed in the production and printing of this book by taking proactive steps such as planting trees in direct proportion to the number of trees used to print books. To learn more about Tree Neutral, please visit **www.treeneutral.com**.

Advantage Media Group is a publisher of business, self-improvement, and professional development books and online learning. We help entrepreneurs, business leaders, and professionals share their stories, passion, and knowledge to help others learn and row. Do you have a manuscript or book idea that you would like us to consider for publishing? Please visit **advantagefamily.com**.

For my kids, Clark, Sam, Zach, Mitch, and McCall,
who are my pride and joy. For my wife, Susan,
who is my inspiration and best friend.

CONTENTS

FOREWORD

CLARK NOTES IN chapter 9, near the end of this book, that one of the things he loves about orthodontic care is "that it works just about 100 percent of the time." *And I agree!* This book explains *why* that is true. It is because orthodontic care involves more than just braces and appliances—as the title, *It's Not About the Braces*, implies. Great orthodontic care requires all the elements that Clark describes: a caring doctor who is properly educated and experienced; a dedicated staff working collaboratively to motivate and energize children, adolescents, and adults; and patients who are flexible and willing to play along to get the results that they are there for. Together, the orthodontist, staff, and patients interact to produce a synergistic environment that just about guarantees success.

Each chapter in this book describes a different aspect of the formula required for producing outstanding patient care, experiences, and outcomes. It starts with having an orthodontist who is rigorously educated to diagnose, plan, and execute high quality treatment—but, more importantly, who is able to look beyond crooked teeth when appropriate, to find other underlying causes and effects. The book is peppered with Clark's interesting stories about individual patients to help to illustrate and personalize his points. This makes each chapter a breeze to read while at the same time driving home the messages he is trying to convey.

One of Clark's most captivating stories involves "Jennifer," an adult patient whose orthodontic experience and outcome was life-changing for her. Braces were something she had wanted for her whole life, and when her husband gave her a Christmas present of orthodontic treatment, she was proud to show off her braces and then to smile broadly when her treatment was completed. Now, she works as a clinical assistant in Clark's office, coaching patients on how to clean and take care of their teeth because braces make that task more difficult to accomplish. As a practicing orthodontist myself, I often recall experiences with specific patients from my past, wondering what happened to them when they grew up and what impact I had on their lives. Jennifer is a perfect example of the powerful influence that being given a healthy, beautiful smile can have on someone's attitude and outlook on life.

As an orthodontic teacher, my greatest sense of satisfaction comes from seeing my students go out into the world independently, have successful careers, and engage in the service of helping others. Clark Andersen was in the very first class that I taught when I joined the faculty of the orthodontic department at Virginia Commonwealth University. There were only three students in that class, so we spent a lot of time working closely together. Since then, I have published numerous scientific research articles, several book chapters, become chair of the orthodontic department and editor of a scientific journal, and lectured all over the world. But this is the first invitation I have received to write a foreword for a book written by one of my former students. It is a great honor, indeed.

In any clinical field—and orthodontics is no exception—one of the most important skills that teachers try to instill in their students is the ability to continue to learn and develop independently, well beyond the time of graduation. Clark's career spanned the early developments of digital technology in orthodontic practice, improvements in the design of braces, introduction of aligners such as Invisalign for treatment, the use of temporary implants, and the recent phenomenon of do-it-yourself (DIY) orthodontics. This book discusses all of these, their advantages and disadvantages, and the truths and myths surrounding them in a very straightforward and practical way. One of my favorite lines of the book explains clearly why DIY orthodontics just doesn't work: because "Every team needs a quarterback" (and "smile-by mail" programs just don't provide one of those—see chapter 7).

This book is a must-read for prospective and new orthodontic patients, parents of patients, and even aspiring and recently graduated orthodontists going out to work with patients on their own for the first time. For patients, it will give you an idea of what to expect, what goes on behind the scenes in the orthodontic office, and the benefits of working cooperatively with a dedicated and caring doctor and staff behind you. For orthodontists, this book will remind you that "It's not (just) about the braces." The personal, story-telling style of the book makes it easy and entertaining to read. There is way more than braces involved in crafting an attractive and healthy smile.

Steven J. Lindauer, DMD, MDentSc
Editor, *The Angle Orthodontist*
Professor and Chair
Department of Orthodontics
School of Dentistry
Virginia Commonwealth University
Richmond, Virginia

INTRODUCTION

YOU COULD SAY I was born to be an orthodontist. In fact, I say it all the time.

My father was an orthodontist, and I grew up in the practice. I started with little chores befitting a small boy, like cleaning, but later I graduated to working in the lab, trimming the plaster models of teeth on a lathe. I found it fascinating, and I marveled at the warm relationship that my dad seemed to have with his patients. Although he's from a different era and practiced in a completely different way than I do today—or even when than I first began practicing—it was always an interesting profession to me, and it never really occurred to me to do something else.

I liked the science and craft required of orthodontics combined with the very rewarding personal interactions my patients and I enjoy, so it gave me a direction in life. I majored in medical biology at the University of Utah and then attended dental school at the Medical College of Virginia, now Virginia Commonwealth University, graduating in 1988.

Would I have become an accountant if my father had been an accountant? Or a lawyer if my father had been a lawyer? We will never know, of course, but I'm glad my life put me on this path, because I cherish the opportunity to make people's lives better every single day.

As a resident dentist at Yale, I saw a patient who had been seen by a periodontist—a dentist who specializes in gum disease and dental implants. After an ordinary cleaning, the patient developed an infection that landed him in the hospital with a brain abscess. It prompted me to research what had gone wrong, and I wrote a paper about the case study that got published in the *Journal of Periodontology*. At that time, little was known about the connection between dental cleanings and the potential for oral pathogens to affect other areas of the body. Today we know that poor oral health is linked to cancer, Alzheimer's, heart disease, and other systemic health issues.

That desire to keep learning more about the science behind oral health, to become as expert as possible, to never stop growing in my profession, has driven me throughout my career and, I hope, made me a better orthodontist today. Any good orthodontist—indeed, any person of science—understands that we are like a shark with respect to our knowledge base: it will cease to be if it stops moving forward.

One other thing happened to me during my dental residency that taught me an important lesson I've carried with me my entire career. This was during the HIV epidemic, when AIDS was still a death sentence, when fear and loathing surrounded the issue and people were afraid of "catching" it from those who were HIV positive.

During that time, postdoctoral students like me provided care in the emergency room. I got called in the middle of the night to examine a man with AIDS for a severe toothache. When I pulled his cheek out to peer into his mouth, the tissue fell away like well-cooked spareribs. His tissue was so compromised that I could look into his mouth and see all the way up to the base of his eyeball. As you can imagine, it was a very scary moment for both of us.

It was clear that this man needed immediate medical care, including an administration of a massive amount of antibiotics to kill the opportunistic bacteria that had invaded his body. At that point in the epidemic, we knew that HIV was carried in bodily fluids like blood. I recognized that there was a small risk of contracting HIV from a blood splash as I inserted an IV needle into a vein, particularly after discovering that the veins in his arms and legs had all collapsed, likely because he was an intravenous drug user. Many other healthcare personnel were reticent to care for this man. But at that moment, my humanity overcame my fear, and I inserted the IV into a vein in his foot.

No one should ever have care withheld from them because of who they are or what they have done in their lives.

Afterward, when I reflected on what had happened, it occurred to me that no one should ever have care withheld from them because of who they are or what they have done in their lives. This man had a mom and a dad and likely other people in his life who loved him. He was not so different from me but for a couple of bad choices and maybe a few bad breaks.

It was an aha moment for me. I knew at that moment that, in my practice, I would never discriminate against any patient, regardless of who they were, what they had done in life, or their ability to pay. I have kept that promise, accepting Medicaid and waiving fees for families in financial distress. This philosophy is even part of the mission statement my staff and I wrote for my orthodontic practice. I count myself lucky to love what I do and have the opportunity to live a full and fulfilling life, and I feel a responsibility to use my gifts to aid those who might not count themselves so lucky.

I know my father would be proud of this choice I have made.

The initial precursors of that lesson were actually planted in my heart during my two-year LDS church mission in a rural Bolivian village so far off the beaten path that they speak the indigenous language Aymara, not Spanish. The people there were so poor they didn't have running water or rudimentary healthcare—but they were happy. In fact, I would say that generally they were happier than most Americans, because they didn't feel anxiety about chasing material wealth. It helped me understand Winston Churchill's prescription for life: "You make a living by what you get. You make a life by what you give."

Knowing that dental school was not my last stop, I returned to the Medical College of Virginia for orthodontic training and a two-year residency after my postdoctoral studies. I did more research there, publishing a paper in the *Journal of the American Dental Association* about how to predict, at an early age, that a patient is susceptible to having an upper canine tooth become impacted in their palate. Identifying this problem years in advance allows us to intervene orthodontically, usually by extracting the baby teeth that stand in the way and will fall out eventually anyway. This revolutionary diagnostic method identifies early those who will likely suffer the impaction. Simply extracting the baby teeth potentially prevents costly and painful surgery, and all their side effects, in those we treat.

I am very proud of that discovery. It followed the path described by Thomas Edison, who said that "genius" is 1 percent inspiration and 99 percent perspiration. What I discovered does not amount to anything in the vicinity of genius; it was the result of following my curiosity, reviewing the current literature, working hard to find revealing data, and applying a solution we found that worked.

I decided to continue working hard and remaining curious about how to improve care for my patients, which is what I've done my entire career. If you were to visit my practice today, you would notice a litany of improvements compared to when I first purchased my father's practice thirtysomething years ago.

It is hard to pinpoint the moment I realized that the science of dentistry and the craft of orthodontics mattered only secondarily in my practice to the art of building relationships with patients and their parents. I don't recall a moment of epiphany so much as a slow recognition, one idea building upon another over time, much the way one builds a sandcastle. One reason I wanted to continue my education beyond dental school was because dentistry often creates a transactional relationship between patient and dentist, particularly between dentists and children who see them once every six months. When I ask my young patients who their dentists are, 90 percent of them do not know. An orthodontist might see a child every few weeks for a year and a half or more. Children who see me do so because they want to—or at least they want to achieve the beautiful smile that will result from our work together. When we are done, a child knows not just the name of the doctor and team of practitioners who fixed their smile but also how they treated them.

The beautiful smile that my team and I create for children (and adults, too, though children comprise about 80 percent of our patients) will last their lifetime and improve their lives in myriad ways beyond just the aesthetic. Our work can alleviate overcrowding, correct a misaligned jaw, relieve inflamed gums, strengthen supporting structures in the jaw, and much more. Speech impediments, headaches, and even bad breath may be corrected with braces.

Seeing a patient of any age walk out the door for the final time with their life changed and a big, beautiful smile on their face is sublime validation for my team and me. If you have ever truly made a significant, tangible improvement in someone's life, you know that feeling of transcendence and gratitude. My team and I often thank our patients, odd as that may seem, because they have afforded us the opportunity to come into their lives and have a positive impact.

After all my dental and orthodontic training, I returned home to my family in Brigham City, Utah, about fifty miles north of Salt Lake City. Family is an artery that runs through the body of my life; I wanted to be close to my parents and siblings then, and I have remained here with my wife to raise five magnificent kids and serve the community that nourished me as a child. Northern Utah is a heavenly slice of the world, with the Great Salt Lake and all the recreational activities it spawns just to the west and the Wellsville and Wasatch Mountains hard against us to the east. It's a skier's, snowboarder's, boater's, fisherman's, hiker's, mountain biker's paradise with four distinct seasons and a great place to raise a family. So this is where I set up shop—or, more accurately, bought my father's shop—and went about building my own reputation.

Orthodontics has, as I have mentioned, offered me tremendous opportunities professionally and personally. It has also opened a window on the public's confusion about the profession, what value it offers to patients, and how it differs from dentistry. Here's how the American Association of Orthodontics puts it:

> The purpose of orthodontic treatment is to create a healthy, functional "bite," which is part tooth alignment and part jaw position. When jaws and teeth line up correctly, they are able to function as nature intended. This promotes oral health and general physical health. That orthodontic treatment also brings about an attractive smile is an added bonus …

Orthodontic treatment will help your child bite and chew, and contribute to clear speech … Self-confidence and self-esteem may improve as orthodontic treatment brings teeth, lips and face into proportion. Straight teeth are less prone to decay, gum disease and injury.[1]

As I embark on my fourth decade of orthodontic practice, I have heard every misconception about my profession you can imagine. The most prevalent misconceptions I hear are these: that a family dentist is also an orthodontist, that the work is all cosmetic, that orthodontic care can't be initiated until after baby teeth have been replaced by adult teeth, that braces are unreasonably expensive and stain teeth, and that sending away for a mold from a faceless company on the internet every few months is a safe and effective way to improve your smile on the cheap.

The internet is a valuable tool and a massive store of information—but it is not particularly good at helping users distinguish valuable information from outright falsehoods. People latch onto a few decontextualized snippets of fact and think they have become informed when in fact they have become misled. This affects every aspect of our lives, and I'm afraid my profession is caught in its jaws. The internet has simultaneously made us vastly more knowledgeable and less informed than ever before.

Consequently, it is no surprise that my patients come to me with questions and misconceptions about how best to promote their oral health and create a beautiful smile. I have attempted to provide honest and forthright information to everyone I meet personally and to spread the truth on our website. It is important to me that people

---

1   "Importance of Orthodontics," American Association of Orthodontists blog, accessed December 11, 2020, https://www.aaoinfo.org/blog/parent-s-guide-post/importance-of-orthodontics/.

have all the information they need to make an informed decision about what to do about their teeth, whether they decide to use my services or not.

Combating myths on the retail level is a losing proposition. Mark Twain said that a lie could travel halfway around the world while the truth is putting on its shoes (although the actual quote predates Twain, whose name wasn't even really Mark Twain—so you see how careful we have to be when gathering information!). That was before there existed instantaneous global communication, which can spread a lie around the world a dozen times before the truth has even turned off its alarm clock. Disabusing people of their misapprehensions one person at a time is not making much of a dent.

That is what has prompted me to write a book. It is a love letter to all the important people in my life—my parents and siblings who molded me into who I am; mentors and teachers throughout my long academic career; my indispensable wife, Susan, and my five children, who have given my life meaning; my team at Edge Orthodontics, who have been instrumental to the success of the practice; and the thousands of patients over the years who have trusted their smiles, or their children's smiles, to me. For the reader, this is designed to be the quintessential orthodontic myth buster—your guide to truth and honesty in service to your teeth, your mouth, and your overall health.

CHAPTER 1

"MY DENTIST IS AN ORTHODONTIST TOO"

A MOTHER I knew well came to us with a daughter in great distress. The fourth of five children, a teenage girl—we'll call her Marie—had been outfitted with braces by someone who was not an orthodontist. This was surprising to me because I had treated her three older siblings and was expecting that if child number four needed orthodontic services, the family would come to our practice.

Well, come to us they did, but in very different circumstances than would have been optimal.

Here's the issue: an orthodontist spends years in a postgraduate orthodontic program and clinical training beyond dental school, learning and practicing the science, craft, and art of repairing dental alignment. At any given time, a million North Americans, mostly children, are equipped with braces to correct their bite, make chewing more functional, and align their teeth for a beautiful smile.

I, myself, passed through the gauntlet of orthodontic school, clinical training, peer-reviewed research, board certification, and now more than thirty years of experience, improving literally thousands of smiles in my Northern Utah communities. (For this book I was asked to estimate how many patients my staff and I have served, and a quick back-of-the-envelope calculation put the number at eight thousand to ten thousand. That astonished us. And then we went back to work.) My staff has decades of experience at my side, ensuring our patients the optimal orthodontic experience. We have learned and grown together, stayed abreast of all the latest advancements, and seen enough "revolutionary breakthroughs" to know which ones have real value and which ones are merely attempts by salespeople to realign the nation's financial balance so that it tilts more steeply toward their own bank accounts.

If you are going to expend the time and money necessary to fit your child with braces, do you want seasoned professionals like me and my team or someone who took a course one weekend?

Let's reframe that question to more vividly illustrate the point. You need a heart transplant. Are you going to have it done by the best cardiothoracic surgeon in the region, the person most experienced in heart transplants, or will you opt to save 20 percent on the price with an internist who attended a seminar on heart transplants at a hotel by the airport?

You need an accountant to handle your complicated tax returns after a foray into business, purchase of property, purchase and sale of complicated securities, amortization, depreciation, and so on. Are you hiring a highly reputable CPA with extra training in these kinds of issues and experience with complex tax returns, or are you trusting your financial well-being to the local storefront tax "specialist," where an accounting student with a week of training in the basics handles your return for a discount price?

I'm guessing you would choose the cardiologist and the CPA, because that is the sensible choice. The mother of this teenager who walked into our practice, after experiencing good results previously with the sensible choice, opted to experiment on her fourth child with the lower-priced alternative. Because we had more important issues to address, I never did ascertain the reasoning. I suppose I also wanted to spare her the embarrassment of discussing what was very clearly an expensive and painful mistake.

Marie was seen by a dentist. Yes, it is legal for a dentist to take a course and become "certified" in orthodontics. Dentists who do this may be sufficiently skilled to handle some simple cases, but it would be almost impossible for such a person, handling just a few orthodontic procedures annually, to acquire the knowledge and skill possessed by me and my ten thousand orthodontic colleagues across the nation. Moreover, were anything out of the ordinary to arise during treatment, which it often does, a dentist would be ill equipped to address it.

Worse, the particular dentist who treated Marie had attended a lecture, perhaps at some luxury resort in Las Vegas, where the purpose of the gathering is a stew of education, networking, socializing, and entertainment—in which the so-called expert, paid by a company selling a product, was advocating for a new kind of treatment that of course employed the company's product. By *new kind*, I mean a kind of treatment for which there is precious little empirical support, if any, and which would horrify all ten thousand of America's orthodontists.

This particular treatment, in a nutshell, involves extracting upper second molars—the wide, flat teeth at the back of the mouth used for grinding food—to avoid future issues with the temporomandibular joint (TMJ), which connects your lower jaw to your skull. There is no evidence that extracting these teeth has any effect on the TMJ. The company advocating this course of treatment proposed that the extraction should be done when braces are affixed.

This dentist returned to his practice armed with this one play in his playbook. As the saying goes, if all you have is a hammer, everything looks like a nail. I'm sure he had the best of intentions, and he might even be a very fine dentist, but he should not be practicing orthodontics, just as operating an automobile each day does not qualify me to be a race car driver.

After two and a half years of ostensible orthodontic treatment, Marie was still wearing braces with no end in sight. She was in pain because, as it turned out, she had an impacted upper, or maxillary, canine tooth embedded in her palate, a problem that would have been revealed with a simple x-ray at the commencement of treatment. The whole situation was a nightmare for this poor teenage girl.

And now it was our nightmare.

Most of our cases start at the beginning and follow a familiar set of time-tested protocols to ensure that each step follows the previous ones logically, building on the progress we have made. We deal with issues as they arise, so that even the most perplexing problems fall into the rubric of care we have developed. It is a formula that has worked for our practice for decades and is probably not significantly different from the methods used by other orthodontic practices.

What almost all our other cases have in common is that we are starting at the beginning. In this case, standards of care had already been breached, and we were forced to attempt to repair egregious errors just to reach the starting line of care. Poor Marie was in for many more months of treatment and the permanent loss of two perfectly functional teeth.

After performing some diagnostic procedures to create a road map for treatment, we removed Marie's braces. That was a relief for her, but unfortunately, further bracing was going to be necessary once we corrected her other problems.

The impacted tooth had to be surgically exposed to allow access to it and to reposition it into its proper alignment. To make room for the canine tooth, sadly, another tooth had to be pulled, making a total of three missing teeth. Imagine being a teenager and suffering the permanent loss of three teeth.

It was a long slog, but we did everything we could to make Marie comfortable, and she supported our efforts with the best possible attitude given the circumstances. The day her braces came off permanently and her beautifully aligned smile gleamed off the mirror was a watershed for her and a relief for her mom. After many heartfelt thank-yous in our office, Marie has continued to express her gratitude by flashing that nearly perfect smile all over town. Her mother has expressed her gratitude by bringing her youngest child to us for orthodontic treatment, her lesson about dentists and orthodontists learned the hard way.

THE DIFFERENCE BETWEEN A DENTIST AND AN ORTHODONTIST

At parties, in casual conversation at the grocery store, and in other informal settings, I regularly hear from people who conflate dentists and orthodontists. As any reputable dentist could tell you, we have different expertise, different areas of knowledge, different educational and training regimens, and different places in the dentofacial treatment continuum. Indeed, many of my referrals come from dentists who recognize the limits of their expertise. Similarly, I would never

To become an orthodontic specialist, a dentist must then earn acceptance into an orthodontic program, which is roughly the equivalent of winning the lottery, except that it is a matter of merit, not luck.

purport to be an expert in crowns, filling cavities, and caring for teeth in that way, although I was trained in the profession alongside today's dentists more than three decades ago. As Marie's case illustrates, we should hire professionals for their specific expertise and not for a discipline with which they have merely a passing familiarity.

Simply put, a dentist is not an orthodontist, though all orthodontists are dentists. If you find that confusing, consider a similar example closer to everyday life: All humans are mammals, but not all mammals are humans. For a mammal to be a human, it must have certain characteristics, like opposable thumbs and an upright gait. For a dentist to be an orthodontist, they must complete further schooling, residency, and often board certification.

All orthodontists go to dental school, complete their clinical training, and earn a doctor of dental surgery degree, just as any dentist does. Most dentists work in a dental office, hospital, or clinic, or they hang out their own shingle. To become an orthodontic specialist, a dentist must then earn acceptance into an orthodontic program, which is roughly the equivalent of winning the lottery, except that it is a matter of merit, not luck.

Consider this: about 50 percent of the college graduates who complete the requirements for dental school admission and take the DAT—the standardized test for acceptance into dental school—are accepted into an accredited dental program, according to Kaplan, the standardized test company. If that sounds too easy, consider that those applying are already a self-selected group of people who know their grades are sufficient to be considered for admittance and have completed all the science requirements, taken the trouble to study for and sit for the standardized test, and gone to the expense of applying for admission. Even then, only half of this select group earns admission to some dental school.

Each year roughly ten thousand college graduates enter dental school, according to Kaplan, but of those who graduate as doctors of dentistry, only three hundred are accepted annually into orthodontic schools. Only the dental students with the highest grades, board scores, and letters of recommendation have any chance of earning a position in a postgraduate orthodontic program. Generally speaking, orthodontists earned grades that put them in the top five of their class in dental school.

In my case, after graduating from Virginia Commonwealth University's medical school cum laude in 1988 as a full-fledged dentist, I entered a postdoctoral fellowship at Yale University's Yale New Haven Hospital. Because of the case I witnessed in which the patient seen by a periodontist—another kind of dental specialist—developed a very dangerous brain abscess, I researched and wrote a paper about the potential for oral pathogens to infect other parts of the body.

After publication of that paper in a dental journal, I returned to Virginia for orthodontic training and a two-year residency. During that time, I published another paper in the *Journal of the American Dental Association* about how to predict whether a child is susceptible to impacted maxillary canine teeth and the benefit of early orthodontic intervention.

I have practiced orthodontics with a great team in Northern Utah for more than thirty years, taking continuing education classes and keeping abreast continually of advances in my field. I do not practice dentistry and have not claimed to be a dentist, even though I have a doctorate in dentistry; in fact, I regularly refer patients to dentists I hold in high esteem in my community for dental care. No dentist could possibly know what I know about orthodontics after years of training and a reputation for excellence fostered by the eight to ten thousand patients we have served in our practice.

YOUR RELATIONSHIP WITH YOUR ORTHODONTIST

It's been said that people don't care how much you know until they know how much you care. Any medical practitioner who deals with people and doesn't treat them with care, concern, patience, and understanding isn't very good at what they do, irrespective of their technical skills. As an orthodontist, I learned decades ago that my scientific knowledge is critical to serving my patients and that expertise at my craft helps me stand out above others in my field, but the single indispensable element that defines a great orthodontic practitioner is treating patients like kings and queens—or, in the cases of the children who make up most of my practice, princes and princesses.

Now, doting on patients and treating them regally does not necessarily distinguish an orthodontist from a dentist. I know many great dentists who are beloved by their patients for their personal warmth, gentle touch, and chairside manner. But imagine bringing your child to the dentist for an annual checkup and returning every few weeks for a year and a half before filling a tooth. By and large, your child will see the dentist once every six months for their checkup, and maybe once or twice besides that to fill a cavity. That is nothing like the intense and sustained relationship the same children develop with their orthodontist, who is delivering a tangible benefit upon completion of treatment. When I ask the children whom I treat the name of their dentist, 90 percent of the time they don't know. Every one of them knows my name, not to mention the names of several of my team members.

Charlie's case demonstrates the relational difference between you and your dentist versus you and your orthodontist.

When I walked into the exam room of my practice, the scene my eyes beheld was not the usual tableau of a family awaiting my arrival for their first encounter with an orthodontist. I often meet nervous children and anxious parents, twirling their hair or gritting their teeth, watching my every move like a hawk. I have met parents who were so ridden with anxiety they talked nonstop and children paralyzed by fear who didn't make a squeak even when I addressed them.

I have become used to all that and have developed an aptitude for putting both children and adults at ease. By displaying confidence in my team's ability to help them, compassion toward their plight, understanding that this may be an overwhelming situation for them, and warmth toward them as individuals, I am almost always able to reduce or eliminate their fear and anxiety. Treating people well is easy if you practice it all the time.

I hire and work with staff who share the philosophy written in our mission statement: to make every patient's visit to us the best part of their day. I have seen them execute this philosophy from the beginning of every patient's visit until they walk out the door. Every day, I walk into exam rooms with confidence that those inside have already been put at ease as much as possible. I also understand that none of the staff members is the orthodontist, the person who is going to put his hands in the patient's mouth and move teeth around. So I am not surprised to see initial discomfort.

This was the first time, though, I had ever encoun-

You can drag the child to the exam chair and make an enemy for life—and probably still fail to get him to open his mouth for any useful examination—or you can take the long view and begin building a relationship with him.

tered a child literally hiding under the table. The patient, a boy of nine or ten years of age whom we will call Charlie, was sitting cross-legged on the floor beneath an exam table and demonstrating no inclination to change that dynamic in any way. As you can imagine, his mother was embarrassed, confused, and even more anxious.

It became clear very quickly that Charlie was not going to budge, and thus a proper exam was impossible. In a case like this, you can drag the child to the exam chair and make an enemy for life—and probably still fail to get him to open his mouth for any useful examination—or you can take the long view and begin building a relationship with him. I chose the latter; since I couldn't bring Mohammed to the mountain, I brought the mountain to Mohammed. That is, I met Charlie where he was—quite literally—by sitting down on the floor with him.

Just imagine you are a ten-year-old boy trying to escape the adult world by dropping to the floor, and the middle-aged orthodontist plops down right there with you! I think my street cred with him skyrocketed with that one small act, particularly because I came as friend, not foe. I was not there to argue with Charlie but to allay his fears and allow him to feel as if he were directing the progress of the appointment.

We had a short conversation about how he felt and why he felt it necessary to hide from us. Frankly, I didn't learn much. If you've ever had a ten-year-old son, you likely know how little you are going to glean from him in an impromptu interview, especially if you're asking him how he feels or why he is acting out. Nonetheless, I listened patiently, hoping to build trust, and asked him if he would do me a favor and just sit in the chair. I promised not to do anything once he was there, just have a conversation while he sits in the chair.

I told his mother that I didn't know what the problem was but promised to be part of the solution and that I was happy to work with her and her son for as long as it took. Taking care of patients' parents is an important part of the job, too, and in this case, it was pretty clear that Mom needed to be reassured as much as Charlie did.

Much to Mom's relief, Charlie got up and climbed into the chair. I walked out of the room for a moment so there could be no doubt in his mind that I was not going to attempt to examine him; then, when I returned, I remained a few feet away and just engaged him and his mom in a three-way conversation, outlining what I planned to do the next time we met, the lack of pain involved, and the long-term benefits of treatment.

When we parted that day, Charlie's mom and I created a plan for Charlie to return every week for the next six months in an iterative process, building his confidence and moving forward one step at a time. As they departed, I told Charlie that it was my expectation that when he returned, he would be ready to sit in the chair and allow me to look inside his mouth. If he did that, I promised, I would not attempt to do anything else but look.

When he returned the next week, he sat in the chair and, after some reticence, allowed me to peer into his mouth—but nothing more. The following week, Charlie sat in the chair, opened his mouth, and allowed me to use a mouth mirror to examine his mouth. Every step of the way, I explained to Charlie and his mother what I was going to do next, why it was important, and how I would use the tool I held in my hand. Over the weeks, I could see Charlie's fears melt away as I made good on every promise and kept him informed every step of the way.

Eventually, Charlie's behavior became cooperative and age appropriate as he learned to trust me. I was able to make a diagnosis and do some minor treatment on him—it turned out he didn't need much orthodontic work, at least not at that point in his life. But Charlie and

I now have a strong bond, one he will likely never have with a dentist, and it may serve us well down the line if he requires more complete orthodontic care as a teenager.

DIAGNOSIS WITH ONE LOOK

You may have heard about the ten-thousand-hour rule, popularized by author Malcolm Gladwell in his best-selling book *Outliers*. The idea is that mastering a skill requires an average of ten thousand hours of dedicated practice, or about an hour and a half per day for twenty years. Whether ten thousand hours is the magic number, or whether it is somewhat more or less, is a subject for debate, but I don't believe there is any serious disagreement over the concept that mastering a discipline requires years of dedicated practice.

I practice orthodontics eight hours per day—give or take—fifty weeks per year and have done so for thirty years, not including my schooling, so by anyone's accounting, I have reached that threshold for mastery. I do not say this to brag, because just about anyone with the background to begin working as an orthodontist and who puts in the sixty thousand hours that I have accumulated over three decades should develop an instinct for it.

That is likely the primary explanation for my ability—I suspect common among experienced orthodontists—to take one look at a person across a room and diagnose in my mind exactly the problem with their smile and the optimal course of treatment to fix it. I can see the position and aspect of the face at ease, its movement during speech, the carriage of the head, and the position of the teeth during smiling and speaking. I might have difficulty articulating it to someone standing next to me, but I can identify and correct any issues.

When you consider an orthodontist, your mind goes right to braces that straighten teeth. That is understandable, as orthodontists do straighten teeth with braces and other appliances. That is the tip of the iceberg, though, like saying a lawyer sues people or an orchestra conductor keeps time. In fact, orthodontics deals with the full diagnosis, prevention, and correction of malpositioned teeth and jaws and is focused on modifying facial growth to alleviate the abnormal alignment of teeth that can lead to an array of health issues, including jaw and head pain, speech impediments, breathing problems, and TMJ disease.

When I see people's faces, I view them through an orthodontic lens. My perspective transcends teeth, because they are a bellwether of health in the musculoskeletal structures around them. Where I might see a smile that suggests an overbite, misaligned teeth, a crowded mouth, jaw and head pain, and sleeping issues, you very likely would not be aware of any physical problems at all. You might simply observe that you are not dazzled by the person's smile. And that would be true even if you were a dentist.

Even confining myself to their smile, I can diagnose smile issues well beyond simply the alignment of teeth. The artistic element of orthodontics attends to much more than straightening teeth; after all, few of us have a straight face or straight lips. The teeth must follow the drape of the lips to present the perfect smile. An experienced orthodontist focuses his attention on the position of the upper lip as it drapes over teeth and the amount of gum showing during a smile.

In fact, most people have an overbite, a word whose meaning is often misconstrued. An overbite is not buck teeth—upper teeth that protrude out beyond the lower teeth. An overbite is a vertical, not horizontal, misalignment in which the upper teeth overlap the top of the lower teeth, narrowing and hiding part of the smile. When ordinary people see someone with an overbite, they don't consciously notice a problem; they are just underwhelmed viscerally. You simply would not think, "Wow, what a great smile!" even if you couldn't articulate why.

An experienced orthodontist will observe diverse issues that affect the smile and dentofacial structures. Here is a case in point: Sometimes I see patients who are wearing the bands on their braces in a way that contravenes the directions for use. This leads to misdirected tension on the teeth, which is not just ineffective but counterproductive. The entire strategy of bracing is to slowly coax the teeth and the palate into the position and shape desired. If the bands are pulling in a direction contrary to the plan or with the wrong amount of tension, they are not doing their job as designed. Misuse of bands undermines the treatment plan and lengthens the amount of time braces must be worn.

All these issues taken together—overbite, curved lips, lip draping, gum visibility, and others—must be taken into account when designing the perfect smile. An experienced orthodontist can see these elements and formulate a basic plan of action at first blush—not that we do it that way. Those ten thousand hours of dedicated practice have equipped practitioners like me to discern instinctively the issues involved and the correct course of treatment. Orthodontic artists, which is to say orthodontists who have the full complement of skills, customize the construction of the smile to the face of each individual patient. If you were to study a perfect smile, you would notice that the top teeth follow the contours of the bottom lip and that the teeth run all the way to the corners of the mouth.

In the next chapter, I will delve more deeply into the role the orthodontist and supporting team play in the patient experience. The most important pieces of equipment in any orthodontist's office—indeed, I imagine, in any healthcare practitioner's office—are the practitioners themselves. Orthodontists work intensely for twelve to twenty-four months or more with their patients—and their parents as well, when the patients are children—at critical times in their physical and emotional development. The nature and intensity of the bond they forge could play a prominent role in that development, for better or worse.

In our practice we believe that it is our responsibility to make a patient's time with us the best part of their day. We don't just believe it, in fact: we announce it. It is part of our mission statement, and we hold ourselves and each other to it daily. For many of our patients, the orthodontist's chair is a place of refuge, where adults are without fail solicitous, loving, understanding, patient, and ever so nice.

Our practice is a place not only where smiles get fixed, but where they are freely shared.

More than the exact style or type of brace, the orthodontic team is the primary determinant of a patient's satisfaction, and I will discuss how in the next chapter.

TAKEAWAYS

→ Hire the right professional for the job. A dentist is not an orthodontist.

→ Orthodontists receive two or three years of added education and clinical training beyond dental school, pass board exams, and specialize in orthodontics. That is a far cry from dentists who take a course and get "certified" in orthodontics.

→ Only the top dental students earn admission to the extraordinarily selective orthodontics programs. Just three hundred new orthodontists are trained annually.

➡ General dentistry and orthodontics concern themselves with different areas of focus, take different perspectives, and have different aims. Don't hire your orthodontist to perform dentistry or your dentist to perform orthodontics on yourself or your family.

➡ Dentists see their patients twice annually for checkups and a couple of times more for procedures. Orthodontists see their patients—generally children—every few weeks for two years. It tends to be a much more intense relationship at a critical period in the child's emotional development.

CHAPTER 2

IT'S NOT ABOUT THE BRACES

DURING MY ORTHODONTIC residency, I was working with the department chairman on an adult patient whose palate was too narrow for his teeth. This is a common problem in orthodontics. A patient comes to us with a malocclusion—literally, bad bite—hoping we can move the teeth into the right position for biting, chewing, and smiling. There is no point in attempting to reposition teeth to achieve this effect if there is no room for them to move, so first in this case, the palate needed to be expanded. Narrow palates are associated with a host of other problems such as mouth breathing and sleep apnea.

The palate—that is, the roof of your mouth—is really two separate plates that fuse together during childhood. The line at which the plates meet is called a suture. If you have had a baby, you know that the same development takes place in their skull, which is one reason we must be very careful with their heads. If you press the center line of a baby's skull, you will feel that it remains soft. In fact, complete fusion of the sutures in the skull doesn't occur until around age twenty-five.

In the palate, the fusing doesn't take quite that long, but as you can imagine, expanding a palate in a child whose suture is not yet completely fused is a lot easier than in an adult whose palate has essentially become one arched bone.

It is not surprising that it was dogma among orthodontists that the roof of a child's mouth can be widened with an appliance that pushes against it over time—known as a palatal expander—but that technique wouldn't work on adults. Most orthodontists recommended adults submit to painful and expensive oral surgery.

My professor and I were considering this option for an adult when I suggested that we try the palatal expander first. Worst-case scenario, it is ineffective, and he has to have the oral surgery anyway. Fortunately, my professor was open to trying something new. Lo and behold, it worked, and our patient avoided having his mouth cut in half.

Most orthodontists were taught in school that this is not an effective treatment, and my impression is that members of my profession generally dismiss palatal expanders for adults out of hand. I'm sure there are adults out there who investigated the possibility of improving their smile and became discouraged when oral surgery was presented as part of the solution.

Because of that early experience, I continued using this appliance and after thirty years still use palatal expanders on adults, many times with great success. In fact, in those decades of practice, the palatal expander has failed to produce the desired result in exactly one case. I would call that empirical proof that palatal expanders can be used successfully on adults. It is proof enough for me and for many happy patients.

The point is that it's not about the tools; it's about the team using the tools. The expander works the same way for every orthodontist, but only an orthodontist who challenges orthodoxy will exploit its utility for all his patients.

That is why I say it's not about the braces.

THE HIDDEN SKILLS OF AN ORTHODONTIST

There are many, many superb orthodontists in America today who are highly skilled at choosing the right braces for a particular circumstance and applying them deftly, to the benefit of their patients. Just to become an orthodontist, as I've already noted, a dentist must distinguish him- or herself among dental school classmates and then spend years in further schooling and clinical training. Then there are the years of experience honing the craft and the continuing education that is absolutely essential as the profession continues to reinvent itself at an ever-accelerating pace.

Moreover, orthodontics is a meritocracy in a way other health professions may not be. When you enter an orthodontist's office, you know exactly the result you desire and expect. You want to walk out of the orthodontist's office at the end of your treatment time with a spectacular smile that lights up the room, and you want to get there with a minimum of pain and suffering.

Any orthodontist who fails to achieve the outcome above with any regularity is going to find him- or herself without patients in no time flat. Because most patients are school-age kids brought in by their mothers, you can imagine how rapidly a couple of bad experiences get shared—especially in the age of instant communication. Unsuccessful orthodontists are like unsuccessful salespeople: they either get good quickly or don't have very successful businesses.

That is not to say that there are not differences in quality among orthodontists. As with any profession, some are more skilled than others. This is a function of raw talent, dedication to the craft, and experience. I am certainly a much better practitioner now entering my fourth decade of practice than I was during my first five years, and I daresay I'm a superior practitioner to just about anyone today in their first five years of practice. That isn't bragging; it is just a matter of experience. If a problem crops up during treatment, as it inevitably does, I have likely seen it before and learned how to solve it.

A skilled practitioner considers not just the present moment but also the future of your smile.

Beyond that, you might not notice the difference between the beautiful smile produced by my treatment and the beautiful smile produced by a less skilled orthodontist—at least at first. Because orthodontics is about much more than aesthetics, as we will explore in the next chapter, you are likely to see the difference over time.

A skilled practitioner considers not just the present moment but also the future of your smile. I am thinking five years down the road to accommodate any adult teeth that have yet to erupt and likely changes in a patient's skeleto-facial structure as they mature.

A skilled practitioner also sees things you don't see. Let me give you an example.

A patient in his thirties whom we will call Gordon came to me with a phalanx of orthodontic issues that ruined his smile and complicated chewing. It was most unfortunate, because otherwise Gordon was a nice-looking man with a good sense of humor. A cross bite affected every one of his thirty-two teeth. None of the top teeth touched their counterparts on the bottom in part because a narrow palate prevented the teeth from lining up correctly. When palate expanders alone failed to correct that issue, I sent him to an oral surgeon to have his suture separated so that palatal expanders could do their job. I won't go into the details of the process, but let's just say that oral surgery is no one's idea of fun. That Gordon would consent to it demonstrates the severity of the problem.

Once we created some room, we used clear aligners to spread his teeth and move them into alignment. After eight months, his front teeth had come forward and Gordon could bite properly. He was delighted and would have been a supremely satisfied customer had I concluded treatment at that point.

Had you looked at Gordon's smile after eight months, the front teeth that comprise the smile were doing their job. You would have judged his smile with a smile of your own. But I knew our work was not done. His back teeth were still not perfectly lined up, so that while he could bite food like the rest of us, chewing would still have been an issue. It was greatly improved, but not perfect, and leaving it that way could have left him with digestion issues as his chewing remained problematic. He might also experience oral hygiene issues because it was difficult to get a toothbrush into all the surfaces.

Gordon's teeth that are visible in his smile had not yet formed into the artistically beautiful smile that my team and I strive for. When we smile, our front teeth do not meet our bottom teeth but cover about the top third of them. On the sides, where our lips curl up during a smile, more of the top teeth and less of the bottom teeth are visible. The orthodontist must account for that and design a smile that fills the opening between our lips aesthetically. It's the sort of thing you might not notice when you look in the mirror for a moment, but people seeing you repeatedly recognize it unconsciously.

We charge a flat fee whether it takes a year or three to achieve the desired result, so all this is in service of perfection, not of increasing fees. Our work with Gordon was not done, and we continued treating him until his teeth were not just improved but magnificent.

He couldn't believe the transformation. "My wife is so happy!" he told us.

This is the level of perfection that truly skilled orthodontists strive for and regularly achieve. It goes far beyond the kind of braces used and speaks instead to the dedication and skill of the practitioner.

WHEN THERE IS ONE ITEM ON THE ORTHODONTIC MENU

There are practitioners in my profession who are wedded to a certain methodology or appliance, whether that is self-ligating braces, Invisalign, universal early intervention, or something else. Many of them are on the speaking circuit, promoting one way of doing things or another, often sponsored handsomely by the company that stands most to benefit from all the new acolytes they accrue. They may be true believers—I don't doubt their sincerity—but they certainly have a vested interest in the concepts they advocate.

To me, this is a little like a police detective investigating a crime and focusing right at the outset on a suspect or theory. Thereafter, they run the risk of unconsciously (or not) interpreting the evidence to fit their preexisting beliefs rather than allowing the evidence to guide them. This is a psychological concept known as confirmation bias, in which we tend to search for, find, remember, and interpret information we find to support our bias and ignore, reinterpret, or forget contradictory evidence. We're all guilty of it, and we're particularly guilty when we have something to gain, financially or emotionally, from our theory being true or to lose from it being false.

An orthodontist with an unhealthy bias toward a particular methodology or concept is more likely to misinterpret information that would lead them away from a suboptimal approach. There are a lot of negatives there, so let me simplify it: they are more likely to steer you wrong, irrespective of their clinical expertise or their artistry in the craft.

It doesn't really matter if they have a financial stake in their preferred method or approach. Research has shown that humans are loath to admit we are wrong about something we have vociferously supported even long after the evidence has debunked it. This is apparent in the "debate" about vaccinations causing autism or allegations that Barack Obama was not born in America, to name just two recent examples. There are those who cling to these shibboleths despite a complete discrediting of the one study linking vaccinations and autism and public release of Obama's birth certificate. I won't go into the psychology of cognitive dissonance here except to say that it results from the damage to our self-image if we are forced to acknowledge that what we espoused passionately and publicly was less than completely true.

If you are putting your smile into the hands of an orthodontist who is driving the train for one approach or another to the exclusion of all others, you are not receiving optimal care. The best approach for you and your very specific requirements might not be the one on that orthodontist's unnecessarily limited menu.

I want to be clear, because I specifically named three popular orthodontic concepts: self-ligating braces, Invisalign, and early intervention, each of which has its uses. I employ all three. Indeed, clear aligners like Invisalign comprise one of the three revolutions in orthodontic care in the last sixty years. As for early intervention, I published a paper in the *Journal of the American Dental Association* even before I became a practicing orthodontist detailing how a particular early orthodontic intervention could prevent serious issues later in childhood. When it comes to my practice, and I would extrapolate this to all orthodontic practices, optimal patient outcomes result from considering all approaches and applying the one that best meets the needs of each individual patient. I can say categorically that there is no one approach that is optimal for everyone.

> **If you think that dealing with young teenagers is difficult— and as a father of five, I know the travails all too well!—imagine the complicating dynamic of dealing with a nervous parent too.**

That is one key delineator between practitioners of orthodontics. The other one has nothing to do with skill at the craft. Let me describe one situation that illustrates how the orthodontist and his team are more important than the type of braces.

Eighty percent of our patients are children under the age of eighteen who have been brought to our offices by their parents. If you think that dealing with young teenagers is difficult—and as a father of five, I know the travails all too well!—imagine the complicating dynamic of dealing with a nervous parent too.

One mother-daughter dynamic was hindering our ability to serve the child, whom we'll call Sabrina to protect her identity. A young teenager, Sabrina was morose during the early checkups. When we asked her a question, her mom always answered, even if the question was about how she felt. We could tell that having her mother hovering constantly was causing anxiety on top of whatever else was bothering her. Moreover, patient feedback is critical during treatment, and we were not getting any.

My team and I conferred and decided that a gentle intervention was necessary. My amazing team of clinicians and administrators, whom I will discuss in more detail later, convinced me that only the orthodontist could carry the message to Mom that she needed to leave the exam room during her daughter's treatment.

Of course, that is not how I put it. Instead, I told Mom an apocryphal story about one of my sons and how he seemed to recede in his parents' shadow until he left for college, during which time he blossomed. Because the teen years are a time of significant emotional transformation, my wife and I wished we had allowed him to spread his wings earlier. I offered a parallel with her situation, reinforcing how this was evidence of deep parental love and concern, and suggested that perhaps our office was a good laboratory for her to give her daughter a chance to grow emotionally while still in the care of adults.

Whew! She was amenable, so we saw Sabrina unencumbered by her mom's smothering love. The result was a completely different child, one who collaborated in her treatment and seemed to enjoy her time in the office. During her time in our care, we could see her confidence growing. Simultaneously, we could see Mom's growing comfort with leaving her daughter alone. I doubt that either was entirely because we had disengaged Sabrina from her mother or even primarily because of it, but we were proud of our role in their improving dynamic, however large or small it might have been. When her course of treatment ended, both Sabrina and her mother thanked us with big smiles. We could see the difference in Sabrina's smile, of course, and also in her self-esteem and her relationship with her mother.

What did the choice of braces have to do with that? The wrong treatment plan for her situation would have prolonged the treatment and perhaps even delivered a slightly less perfect smile. It wouldn't have changed our relationship with Sabrina, her emotional growth, or her mother's.

THE BEST PART OF YOUR DAY

The mantra at our practice is that we want the visit to the orthodontist to be the best part of every patient's day. That means from the moment a patient walks in the door to the moment they leave, everyone they encounter is warm, doting, and understanding. The culture in our practice is built around this concept; indeed, we meet first thing each morning and reinforce to each other how we are going to execute that idea. We trade information about the issues in patients' lives and who might need a little extra TLC today. In almost every case, it is a member of the team, not I, who shares this bit of intelligence.

Each of us makes a commitment to each other that we are going to put a smile on every patient's face even before we fix that smile. We are going to put a smile on every parent's face. We are going to do everything we can to make our patients feel like guests at a five-star hotel and to make their time at our office the best part of their day.

Keep in mind that 80 percent of our patients are children, most of them in their teen years. This is a time fraught with emotional baggage, raging hormones, perverse peer pressure, and increasing expectations. I experienced these things as a teenager eons ago, and that was long before the added burden of social media presenting highlight reels of everyone else's life for comparison. In many cases, the youngsters who enter our practice have been buffeted by psychological stressors all day, and the same is in store for them tomorrow. They come to us worried, stressed, and anxious.

Given that, we work to make our office an oasis for them, a place where only nonjudgmental people who care about their physical and emotional well-being do nothing but make them feel good every minute they are with us.

Not only are our patients treated like princes and princesses in our offices, but something good is happening to them. While the kids at school belittle them for issues with their teeth; while malocclusions cause them pain, difficulty breathing, or chewing; whatever the problem associated with their teeth, here we come to wash it all away. I know that kids get mocked for wearing braces, too, but at least they know that they are moving in a positive direction toward a brighter, more pleasing smile.

To put children and their parents at ease right from the start, I get off my high horse. I am Dr. Andersen when they walk in the door, but I ask everyone to call me Clark. Moms, dads, thirteen-year-olds all call me Clark. My staff calls me by my first name and refer to me that way. The only patient I've ever had who didn't call me by my first name was my son. He called me Dad.

Being known by my first name demystifies the orthodontic experience. Children don't see me as some great wizard commanding the complex operation that will be taking place in their mouth but as a kindly adult who is one of a team of people taking care of them. If a patient—or even a parent—has a question or a complaint, it might seem impertinent to dare question Dr. Andersen. But it's easy to wonder aloud to Clark.

Just try saying each of these out loud, and see how it feels:

"Why do I have to keep this on all the time, Dr. Andersen?" It sounds like a challenge of some important person's authority, doesn't it?

"Why do I have to keep this on all the time, Clark?" sounds like two folks kicking around an idea.

Whenever a child asks a question about their care, I always respond, "That's a great question. I'm glad you asked," before launching into my answer. I want everyone in the chair and beside it to feel comfortable about every step of the process. To be honest, I don't get a lot of these questions, because I'm always teaching as I proceed, walking the patient and whomever is accompanying them through each step of the process. This relieves anxiety and makes them feel like part of the process.

Of course, most patients spend less time with me than they do with my staff. Members of my team greet everyone when they walk in the door, complete their intake, prep them for care, handle the financial arrangements, and book future appointments. If the people I work with weren't among the kindest and warmest people, it wouldn't matter how nice I was.

It probably won't come as a surprise that my assistants and administrative staff have generally been with me for a long time. Our office is a place of bonhomie that happens to dabble in orthodontics. If you listened to the chatter in our office, you would hear a lot more talk about football teams, college alma maters, high school proms, weekend plans, and neighborhood gossip than about teeth, and most of that conversation is initiated by the people I have the honor and pleasure of working with. We truly have fun together because we are all so rewarded by the joy we bring to our patients' lives. We all truly believe that our patients are doing us a service by allowing us to brighten their days.

In fact, most of my staff were patients before they were employees. They enjoyed the experience so much that they agreed to bring their skill set to our office. We all feel very blessed to work together, and I think that patients can see and appreciate that.

As I mentioned, most of our patients are teenagers, often ridden with angst. We take seriously the idea that we are treating so much more than teeth, so long before we examine their teeth, we delve into their state of mind. I don't even pick up an instrument until after I have asked my patients about their day, their life generally, their hopes and dreams, their preferences and desires, and their fears and concerns as well. I want to be able to make some reference to their preferred activities, their favorite school subjects, or the teams they follow. I want to be sensitive to their anxieties and tuned in to their state of mind that day.

Because, as you already know, I'm working to make sure their time with us is the best part of their day.

ABIGAIL NEEDED TENDERNESS MORE THAN BRACES

Take the case of Abigail, a thirteen-year-old with some serious dental issues whose demeanor when she came to us could make you cry. Abigail was so glum when she arrived at our office the first time, one couldn't be blamed for feeling that she was a miserable kid. And she was miserable, in the sense that she was deeply unhappy. She wouldn't look at me or talk to me or engage with any of us. We could see that her mom was embarrassed by her affect but resigned to it simultaneously. It seemed to me upon meeting them that Abigail wasn't acting like this; she was sad all the time.

It doesn't take a psychologist to understand that a child who appears to be constantly on the verge of tears, particularly when people are being so nice to her, is seriously hurt. I realized at that moment that Abigail didn't need an orthodontist so much as a therapist. Well, I'm not a therapist, but I am a dad who was highly engaged in the raising of his children, and I know what a father's incomparable love feels like. Abigail stoked my paternal instincts and touched my heart. So I did something very important early in our meeting: I put aside the tools of my profession, pulled up a chair at Abigail's level, took her hand and just started talking to her. I asked about her day and about her school experience. I gave her space to answer and let silence hang in the air when she didn't immediately respond. I never mentioned the word *braces*.

It took Abigail a while, but little by little she began to open up. She revealed how bullied she felt at school, in part because of her teeth.

> **For Abigail, the orthodontist's office became a place where she could share how she felt in a cocoon of unconditional affection.**

She divulged how few friends she had, how she often ate lunch alone, and how she felt like an outcast. Her mother expressed shock at these revelations, none of which Abigail had communicated to her. Abigail wasn't mean or taciturn; she was just lonely and depressed.

My clinical assistant and I listened and cooed and made it clear that we understood and empathized with her pain. We matched our demeanor and tone to hers. And we encouraged her to keep talking. Neither of us ever made a move toward our instruments. For Abigail, the orthodontist's office became a place where she could share how she felt in a cocoon of unconditional affection.

Thereafter, every time Abigail arrived, the staff would find opportunities and excuses to introduce her to some other teen in the waiting room or the office. If we had a patient who went to her school, we would mention them to her so perhaps she would have something in common to discuss with that child in the lunchroom or the classroom the next day.

Obviously, we couldn't cure all the issues in Abigail's life, and she wasn't magically gregarious and joyful the next session. We did observe her engaging in hushed conversation with other teenage girls in the waiting room, and she did quickly become more trusting and communicative. As treatment proceeded, she could see how her teeth were becoming straighter. I believe she was beginning to visualize herself as a more attractive person, and that may have buoyed her spirits.

By the time her treatment was concluded, Abigail's affect was unexceptional, and she smiled ... occasionally. In fact, she comes back to visit periodically and honors us with big, resplendent smiles.

What kind of braces did we use to repair Abigail's multiple orthodontic issues? I don't remember. That's not really the point. What distinguished her experience was that in the midst of severe emotional distress, her orthodontist's office was a sanctuary where the entire staff listened and understood. And gave her a beautiful smile.

It's just not about the braces.

It isn't about the braces for Kimberly, a woman who brought children to us for treatment and was so highly satisfied with the experience that she decided she needed to fix her own smile when the time came to get braces for her nephew. There was just one problem: Kimberly had moved to central Wyoming, a six-hour car ride away.

Ordinarily, our office is open Monday through Friday, giving the staff and me time off on weekends for a reasonable work-life balance. We work hard during the week, putting service to our patients above all, but it is important that we all enjoy our families and surroundings as well. We live in a beautiful part of the world on the edge of the Wellsville and Wasatch Mountains and beside the northern edge of the Great Salt Lake.

For Kimberly and her nephew to see us during the week would have required taking two days off from work and school, one to drive down to us and receive treatment and another one to return home. For almost everyone but retired people, this is an untenable arrangement. The obvious accommodation was for us to open on Saturdays just for them. It would mean half a day of work on our off day.

So that is what we did. In fact, we've done that dozens of times, because if it's not about the braces, it had better be about an orthodontist's office that flexes to meet the needs of its customers. Such treatment doesn't require the complete staff—just me alone or me and an assistant—and the occasional six-day work week is a small price to pay for the reward of seeing a woman and her nephew smile. I'd like to think that we're enlightened in that way, but we're honest enough with ourselves to recognize it as enlightened self-interest, because the long-term effect of accommodating patients like Kimberly is that she remains loyal to us and continues to bring her family to us for treatment, passing dozens of orthodontists along the way to get to our office. The ratio of goodwill engendered to sacrifice made is off the charts, enough that it's sometimes a wonder to me how many retail operations fail to grasp this simple concept.

We were looking for that smile when we took off Kimberly's braces and held up a mirror to her, but boy, were we in for a shock. She didn't smile at all; instead, she burst into tears. I thought we had provided her with an artistic smile that would enhance her self-esteem and was mortified by her reaction, steeling myself for the stream of invective that I thought was inevitably to follow. When she finally contained her sobs, she told us that she had wanted this her whole life. I guess I have to work on my ability to distinguish tears of sadness from tears of joy. It added the final vindication to my decision to cut my weekend in half every month or so for a loyal customer.

WHEN THE BRACES DON'T MATTER AT ALL

We had one patient, twelve-year-old Patrick, suffering from a severe case of ectodermal dysplasia—a group of disorders that create abnormalities of the skin, sweat glands, hair, teeth, and nails. Among

Patrick's symptoms was a random jumble of teeth, about half the normal number and pointing in every direction at once. Patrick's ability to bite, chew, and smile were all compromised, and as a result, he was at high risk for digestion and hygiene issues.

Working in an interdisciplinary arrangement with a dentist and prosthodontist—a specialist in creating false teeth—our office's role was to straighten Patrick's existing teeth while leaving room for new teeth to be implanted. This was a challenging endeavor because braces that pull teeth into the correct position are normally anchored to the teeth, which in this case didn't exist. The course of treatment included taking plastic teeth, reshaping them to fit in Patrick's mouth, and gluing the braces to them.

Our purpose right now in Patrick's treatment regimen is to provide temporary functional ability to bite and chew. Ultimately, as his baby teeth fall out, he is going to need dental implants. Our involvement will require years of patience and persistence and will not be profitable from a monetary standpoint, but that is hardly the point. The point is to give this kid some kind of normal life now and in the future.

TAKEAWAYS

➡ There are a variety of ways to brace and move teeth, each of which has its own set of advantages and disadvantages.

➡ Any orthodontist who limits him- or herself to one kind of bracing system is doing the customers a disservice. Even those who evangelize a particular type tend to see all orthodontic issues through that one prism and are denying their patients the full option set.

→ Much more important than which kind of braces an orthodontist uses is the orthodontist and his or her staff. Patients should pay more attention to the skill and experience of the orthodontist.

→ Orthodontists work primarily with young teens and their anxious parents, so kind, patient practitioners and staff are much more important than the type of braces they use.

→ Look for an orthodontist who is flexible too. Do they accept payment plans and make provisions for special cases?

CHAPTER 3

"ISN'T IT JUST COSMETIC?"

FROM TIME TO TIME I get this question from fathers who are dubious about spending a few thousand dollars to fix their children's teeth. This question is usually issued as a challenge, as in, "Come on, isn't all this merely cosmetic?" Even before addressing the false assumptions in this question, I wonder whether Dad asks the same question of his wife's hairdresser about her monthly hair appointments or the clothing store about his business suit. How about his son's overpriced sneakers, his daughter's designer jeans, or all the makeup his wife purchases over the course of a year? Isn't all that merely cosmetic?

In fact, we spend a lot of money every year to make ourselves look good and nothing else, and I'll bet none of the fathers who query me ever consider those other purchases optional.

In the United States today, and probably everywhere in the world, for better or worse, looks matter. Study after study has found that physically attractive people are viewed as more intelligent, honest, and capable.[2] People considered physically attractive perform better in business and in social situations. Companies with better-looking executives have higher revenue and profits. Studies have even discovered that newborns react more positively to people considered by adults to be physically attractive.

In one study of many with a similar theme, beauty and income were linked, with physically attractive men and women earning thousands of dollars more annually than ordinary-looking people.[3] Good-looking people are hired sooner, get promotions more quickly, and enjoy job perks like travel and tickets to events more often than others.

The reasons for this are varied and far beyond my area of expertise, so I will simply summarize what the experts say. Physical beauty suggests vigor and strength along with the ability to procreate successfully. Our ancient progenitors sought out the best candidates to pass on their genes and so were naturally inclined toward those of the opposite sex possessing those qualities. Although that is significantly less important in modern society, virtually every element of public life favors beauty and encourages all of us to seek it in ourselves and others. Advertising and marketing particularly, because they are the business of creating need, bombard us with messages that suggest we are incomplete or unworthy unless we achieve unattainable levels of beauty.

To give one example of how this can deform a society, one of three women aged nineteen to twenty-nine in South Korea today has had some kind of facial surgery for purely cosmetic reasons. The Huff-

---

2   See, for instance, Yoann Lopez et al., "Influence of Teeth on the Smile and Physical Attractiveness. A New Internet Based Assessing Method," *Open Journal of Stomatology* 3 (2013): 52–57, http://dx.doi.org/10.4236/ojst.2013.31010.

3   Daniel S. Hamermesh and Jeff E. Biddle, "Beauty and the Labor Market," National Bureau of Economic Research, November 1993, https://www.nber.org/papers/w4518.

ington Post reports that it is not uncommon for South Korean high school girls to receive plastic surgery as a graduation present from their parents. South Koreans explain this phenomenon as being part of the national obsession for growth and self-improvement, not as a need to increase beauty for beauty's sake.

If television was the driving force behind these messages in the previous fifty years, today it is social media. Behavioral scientist Clarissa Silva found that 60 percent of adults say they feel worse about themselves as a result of using social media.[4] Experts point out that many of the exemplars of beauty that we see in popular media are airbrushed, photoshopped, and otherwise distorted to conform with cultural notions of beauty. Models weigh, on average, 23 percent less than the average woman. This raises the beauty bar

Part of the benefit of orthodontic care is that it creates near-perfect symmetry of the teeth, which generally conveys this characteristic to the entire mouth.

to unreachable levels and deepens the self-esteem issues experienced by the most vulnerable populations—like teenagers.

According to research by Dove, the soap company owned by Unilever, nearly three-quarters of girls aged fifteen to seventeen have skipped school or avoided other normal daily activities that involve interactions with people because they feel bad about their looks.

In many of the studies, the measure of physical attractiveness is based on facial symmetry—how closely the left side of the face mirrors the right side of the face. This has been demonstrated to correlate with

---

4   Clarissa Silva, "Social Media's Impact on Self-Esteem," HuffPost, February 22, 2017, https://www.huffpost.com/entry/social-medias-impact-on-self-esteem_b_58ade03 8e4b0d818c4f0a4e4.

our perception of beauty, with evolutionary roots that signal robust health and genetic quality.[5] Part of the benefit of orthodontic care is that it creates near-perfect symmetry of the teeth, which generally conveys this characteristic to the entire mouth.

So when parents ask me, "Isn't this just cosmetic?" I say facetiously, "Yes, and if you want your child to get married and move out of your house, you'll get them braces."

Consider the downside of not making these purchases that are "merely cosmetic." Most of our patients are twelve to sixteen years old, right in the sweet spot of a crucial developmental stage physically and emotionally. They spend most of their days in a cauldron of peer pressure and raging hormones facing the unfiltered judgment of their peers. Young teenagers value fitting in above all else, eschewing anything that makes them look or seem different. Nothing screams "tease me" or "bully me" like being unusual in junior or senior high school. With respect to orthodontic issues, it can lead to being called some variation of "bucktooth." Between one-quarter and one-third of American teenagers report that they have been bullied, with being perceived as "different" rated the number one risk factor.

That, of course, is an analog view of adolescence. Today's teens live in a digital world where mocking goes far beyond the school corridor and into the ether for the entire universe to see. In the most extreme cases, teenagers facing heartbreaking harassment from peers on social media have committed suicide. I don't mean to be melodramatic, since this is obviously an anomalous worst-case scenario. I am not arguing that a pair of sneakers or orthodontic work to straighten teeth is lifesaving. I am simply putting the concept of cosmetic improvements in

---

5   Gillian Rhodes et al., "Facial Symmetry and the Perception of Beauty," *Psychonomic Bulletin & Review* 5 (1998): 659–669, https://doi.org/10.3758/BF03208842.

the context of a teenager's life, where the highest order of happiness is contingent on social acceptance.

The research around social media is sobering and dishearten-ing. Use of social media has been linked to loneliness, envy, anxiety, depression, and decreased social skills. Because others on social media present a sanitized view of their lives, each of us compares our whole life experience to only the best moments of our "friends."[6]

This has proved difficult for adults and nearly impossible for the half-developed psyches of teenagers. Studies from the University of Pittsburgh, among many others, found that teenagers' use of social media correlates with negative body image, eating disorders, sleep deprivation, and depression, that it exacerbates loneliness and reduces satisfaction with life.[7] At the most awkward time of life, the last thing today's teens need is to look "funny" by the standards of their peers.

We will get into this more in the next chapter, but we have even encountered children who come to our office begging for braces so they can be like their school comrades. Sometimes we have to convince them—and even occasionally their parents—that there is no point in bracing baby teeth when they are just going to fall out and they will have to return for braces on their adult teeth. These young teens and preteens are so desperate to fit in that they are willing to endure the application of appliances on their teeth for a year or two even absent any efficacy.

---

6   Maria Konnikova, "How Facebook Makes Us Unhappy," *New Yorker*, September 10, 2013, https://www.newyorker.com/tech/annals-of-technology/how-facebook-makes-us-unhappy.

7   Jaime Sidani et al., "The Association between Social Media Use and Eating Concerns among US Young Adults," *Journal of the Academy of Nutrition and Dietetics* 116, no. 9 (September 2016): 1465–1472, https://doi.org/10.1016/j.jand.2016.03.021; Jessica Levenson et al., "Social Media Use Before Bed and Sleep Disturbance Among Young Adults in the United States: A Nationally Representative Study," *Sleep* 40, no. 9 (September 1, 2017): https://doi.org/10.1093/sleep/zsx113.

On the flip side, we regularly observe young patients in our office taking selfies while in the chair getting braces. Becoming part of the braces crowd, joining the tribe of kids wearing braces, qualifies for the documentary footage of their life. I sometimes wonder whether they would be happy with placebo braces that didn't actually straighten their teeth, just so long as they could get their membership card in the club.

Are braces just cosmetic? No, but even if they were, don't dismiss the extreme importance in modern American society of looking good. It is not an extravagance but a critically important part of everyone's life. I daresay that most adults in America today who grew up middle class or above—I don't know of any research on the subject—would wish their parents had spent a few thousand dollars on them as adolescents to improve their visage and add to their lifetime earning potential and all the other benefits of added beauty.

ORTHODONTICS IS WAY MORE THAN AESTHETICS

We have a young man in treatment as I write these words whose condition is a long-term health issue that requires orthodontic intervention. Teddy's father not only would never challenge our work as merely cosmetic but is very eager for us to help his son.

Teddy was born with a cleft palate that was repaired when he was a small child. It left him with the telltale cleft lip and an extreme underbite at fourteen years of age. An underbite means that his lower front teeth protrude beyond his upper front teeth. Underbites can cause serious functional and cosmetic issues. On the aesthetic side, underbites give that "bulldog" appearance, particularly in the case of a severe underbite where the lower teeth protrude far out beyond the upper set. When Teddy smiles, his front teeth can't be seen, giving him a toothless look. It is really quite heartbreaking.

Even if this were the only issue, Teddy and his father would be keen to have it repaired. A fourteen-year-old boy with a serious underbite is headed for a high school career filled with scorn and loneliness, not to mention a life without dates. Indeed, when I asked him what one thing he wanted most from treatment, he said, "I want front teeth." For him, the merely cosmetic is the most important benefit of orthodontic treatment, because he understands from hard experience that aesthetics affect every aspect of his life.

If that weren't disturbing enough, significant underbites like Teddy's can cause difficulty biting and chewing food, challenges articulating words, and potential pain from a misaligned jaw. That misalignment can lead to TMD—disease of the temporomandibular joint, where the lower jaw meets the face below the ears. There are a host of foods—corn on the cob and whole apples jump to mind—that he almost certainly has never been able to eat. He would have to remove the corn from the cob and cut the apple into small pieces to have any hope of consuming them. How inclined would you be to eat an apple if one of its signature benefits—that it is highly portable and requires no preparation—was lost to you?

A person whose food choices are significantly limited and who can't properly chew

Failing to chew increases the likelihood of choking and burdens the stomach and the rest of the digestive tract.

their food is at higher risk for a whole host of digestive and nutritional problems as well. Failing to chew increases the likelihood of choking and burdens the stomach and the rest of the digestive tract, which are forced into compensating for the early stages of food breakdown that ordinarily occur in the mouth. Good chewing increases nutrient intake, reduces bacteria buildup, and cuts the risk of food poisoning. Clearly, the problems with Teddy's teeth could easily cascade throughout his body.

Imagine entering high school with a distorted facial presentation, difficulty being understood by teachers and classmates, physical jaw pain, and problems eating food. That is one tough row to hoe—and it wasn't Teddy's only problem.

Teddy also suffered from a mouthful of teeth that pointed higgledy-piggledy in every direction. Consequently, while he is challenged to bite hard food, he is almost completely unable to chew with his molars and premolars—the back teeth we all use to masticate. If his teeth were street signs, you wouldn't know whether to head north, south, east, or west. I don't mean to make light of Teddy's condition, because his first fourteen years had to have been a psychological and physiological minefield. As a dad, I sympathized with both Teddy and his father.

I think it is worth mentioning in Teddy's case that despite all the hardship he has endured, he has a remarkable outlook on life. He has never once complained or pitied himself; he is friendly and outgoing to the extent that a young man unable to flash a real smile can be. I can already tell that Teddy is going to become a staff favorite in no time.

The plan of attack in this case is complex and long term. Teddy is going to spend so much time with us that he and I are bound to become bosom buddies. The course of treatment for more common conditions is about eighteen months from first appointment to last, but Teddy will still be with us well into his junior year of high school and maybe his senior year as well. The good news is that when we are done treating him, his whole life is going to be upended. He will be able to bite and chew like a normal person and flash a toothsome smile that lights up the room. I can't wait to begin fixing his myriad issues and seeing the transformation in this teen. It is going to be nothing short of life changing for him and deeply rewarding for our entire team.

OTHER FUNCTIONAL ISSUES

Orthodontists commonly treat the very opposite problem—an overbite. An overbite is not what you think; it is not necessarily buck teeth. *Buck teeth* is what orthodontists call an overjet, and it involves a horizontal misalignment of the top and bottom front teeth. An overbite is a vertical misalignment—that is, when the bottoms of the upper front teeth cover too much of the top of the lower front teeth.

Is that confusing? Think of it this way: When we smile, all our upper front teeth should be visible. An overbite occurs when the upper teeth mostly or completely cover the lower teeth.

This is a cosmetic issue, of course, but also a functional issue. In a deep overbite, the upper teeth can contact the lower gums repeatedly, causing recession of the gums and gum disease. The lower teeth may be doing the same to the gums at the back of the upper teeth. People who ignore a deep overbite and continue this process often wear down their top teeth by their forties. By then, the level of erosion of the teeth may preclude any attempt by a dentist or an orthodontist to reverse the damage, because the antidote to an overbite is to use braces of one type or another to coax the teeth into the correct position. Once adults have worn away their teeth, there is nothing on which to anchor the braces.

A NOTE ON TMJ PAIN

Studies have found a significant correlation between an overbite and TMD—dysfunction in the temporomandibular joint, causing pain and possibly wearing down of the joint. TMD issues are so vexing for doctors that most health insurance companies don't cover TMJ surgery. It is important for me as an orthodontist to mention here that an important study by the National Institutes of Health has demonstrated that correcting the alignment of teeth does not improve the TM joint or ease TMD, nor is there any reciprocal relationship.[8]

Malocclusions and TMD do not appear to cause each other but may be associated by a common parafunctional imbalance. That is, things like grinding or clenching teeth, trauma from an accident, or some other independent variable may cause TMD and a malocclusion, but fixing one has not been shown to have any effect on the other. Nor, says the study, are orthodontic treatments responsible for the occurrence of TMD.

No credible medical professional in any discipline should be in the business of charging people for treatment that the medical literature has concluded is ineffective.

I'll pause for a moment here to note once again the multisyllabic orthodontic word I have introduced: *malocclusion*. This literally means "bad bite" and is a catchall term for the pathologies we will be discussing in this book.

One winter, the mother of a patient was in a car accident, and the next time she accompanied her child to our office, she complained

---

8   James A. McNamara Jr., "Orthodontic Treatment and Temporomandibular Disorders," *Oral Surgery, Oral Medicine, Oral Pathology and Oral Radiology* 83, no. 1 (January 1997): 107–117, https://doi.org/10.1016/S1079-2104(97)90100-1.

that her teeth were not fitting together correctly. I examined her and found swelling in the jaw, so I prescribed anti-inflammatories, hoping the reduced swelling would resolve the issue. I didn't hear from her and so assumed all was well. This is the orthodontist's equivalent of "Take two aspirin and call me in the morning."

Five months later she returned with the complaint renewed after accidentally getting hit in the jaw at home. The swelling in her jaw appeared minimal, leaving me stumped.

Because of the empirical evidence now facing my profession, one thing I was not going to do was recommend any orthodontic treatment. No credible medical professional in any discipline should be in the business of charging people for treatment that the medical literature has concluded is ineffective. I have talked to practitioners in other fields who have confided that they treat patients for symptoms that time alone will heal, knowing that their intervention has little to do with the resolution of the issue. Their patients feel better and attribute it to their treatment.

Even were I convinced that my stature among patients would grow by the application of such treatment, I would decline, and I imagine most orthodontists—indeed many if not most other health-care professionals—would agree. A doctor without integrity is a charlatan, and a dangerous one at that.

Instead, I examined the relationship of her teeth and noticed that one upper tooth was more heavily contacting a lower tooth and preventing full contact of her back teeth. I smoothed down the offending tooth ever so slightly and—voila!—she reported instant and complete relief. The treatment took all of three minutes and required all the expertise of a good diagnosis.

Treatment of an overbite is best done in childhood when the structures of the jaw are still developing and more pliable. It usually involves a growth modification device to help position and expand the jaw, braces to move the teeth slowly back to their correct position, and a retainer to keep the new alignment of teeth in place. This process usually takes about eighteen months from the very first appointment to the very last and requires a certain level of discipline on the part of the patient. For example, they must be careful to clean their teeth and the braces assiduously, they must wear the retainer exactly as indicated, and they must come for all their appointments.

OVERJETS, BUCK TEETH, AND THEIR SERIOUS IMPLICATIONS

Vertical overbites are often accompanied by overjets—which are really horizontal overbites—and result in buck teeth. Our upper front teeth ordinarily protrude about two millimeters, or about a tenth of an inch, beyond our lower teeth. That is hardly perceptible. Orthodontists become involved when the disparity between the upper and lower teeth is greater than that. I have seen patients whose uppers protrude ten or twenty times the optimal amount.

Besides creating a malformation of the mouth that invites derision, buck teeth can inhibit chewing, cause speech impediments, and create airway concerns. Buck teeth result from a narrow arch in the mouth, a protruding upper jaw, a receded lower jaw, and thumb- or finger-sucking habits, all of which impact the airway. Narrow airways cause snoring, sleep breathing disorder, and sleep apnea. Children with buck teeth also face a sharply higher risk of trauma to their top front teeth. The same way that getting hit in the face is most perilous to the nose, which sticks out beyond any other facial feature, getting hit in the mouth presents danger to the front teeth if they are protruding well beyond the normal position.

Buck teeth are most often corrected with braces to move the teeth and jaws into improved alignment. A palatal expander may also be used in those cases where the malocclusion is accompanied by a narrow palate, crossbite, or crowding in the mouth.

A word about braces here: I use the term as an umbrella for all the various types of systems that realign teeth. Classical brackets, bands, and wires are one form of braces and remain the standard. Self-ligating braces replace the rubber bands and metal ties with small metal doors, clear braces made of porcelain or other aesthetic materials, and even lingual braces placed on the tongue side of the teeth. Clear aligners, best known by the brand name Invisalign, are plastic trays that fit over the teeth and move them from the starting position into an intermediate position. A new aligner is then worn to move the teeth to the next phase, and so on.

With any bracing system, the expertise of an orthodontist is required to determine which bracing system is optimal for a particular pathology and patient.

These different systems have their various advantages and disadvantages. Clear aligners work in most but not all situations and require the compliance of the patients, since they can be removed. Self-ligating braces have their value, but some of their benefits are overblown and not worth the significant added cost. As with any bracing system, the expertise of an orthodontist is required to determine which bracing system is optimal for a particular pathology and patient.

CROSSBITES AND FENCE POSTS

Another common dental issue treated by orthodontists is the crossbite. As I mentioned, when teeth are in their proper position, the top teeth sit about two millimeters outside the bottom teeth. A crossbite exists when one or more top teeth are overlapped by lower teeth, just the opposite of the normal relationship. This misaligned bite can occur anywhere in the mouth—in the front, sides, or back—and cause difficulty chewing, uneven tooth wear, gum recession, and other issues. Severe crossbites, which is what I described in Teddy's case, where his teeth pointed in every direction at once, can even lead to jaw, neck, and shoulder pain and are also aesthetically displeasing.

Think of a tooth as a fence post. In a crossbite, the tooth may be pointing sideways or positioned wrong, and as a result it is banging into or rubbing against other teeth during chewing. That's the equivalent of taking that fence post and wiggling it in the ground. At the outset, the post is solidly grounded, but over time it will become looser and looser. That is the effect of a crossbite on misaligned teeth.

As with all orthodontic issues, posterior crossbites are best treated in childhood or adolescence with palatal expanders and braces that gently guide the teeth over time into the correct position and orientation. As with other orthodontic issues, waiting until adulthood presents a whole host of preventable issues and complicates the treatment. It can even reduce its efficacy in some cases.

In all these cases, although there is a cosmetic component to straightening teeth, the primary purpose is to reposition teeth, jaw, and palate for optimum biting, chewing, swallowing, and breathing. The recounting I have made here of health issues addressed with orthodontic treatment is merely a summary of the most common; patients who have received treatment will testify to a host of other functional benefits that followed their time in our care.

Orthodontists perform another service that is beyond the scope of their treatment regimen: they assess oral structures and can diagnose issues treated by other specialists. For example, because of an orthodontist's expertise in the oral space, he or she can spot issues that might affect the airway, as we have discussed. An orthodontist can recognize any airway issues that may negatively impact development and recommend an evaluation for a tonsillectomy and adenoidectomy or can potentially correct the problem with the use of a palatal expander to open the upper palate, which also serves as the nasal floor.

Treatment for this purpose is usually performed in conjunction with other specialists like ENTs or allergists.

Airway issues are often associated with mouth breathing, which has been found to change the shape of the face over time, creating long, narrow faces and mouths, gummy smiles, and dental malocclusions, including crowded teeth and open bites—where the teeth don't meet. Intervening on airway issues early can cascade into preventing orthodontic issues down the road. That creates a virtuous cycle of orthodontic treatment to address airway issues by widening the palate that ultimately reduces later orthodontic issues.

One issue we see a lot, and one that we will consider in more detail in the next chapter, is adult teeth that erupt before the baby teeth have fallen out. Without a place to emerge, the adult teeth poke out through the gums oriented in random directions. These cases require the removal of baby teeth—what dentists call primary teeth, as opposed to permanent or adult teeth—and orthodontic treatment to corral the wayward permanent teeth into their correct position and alignment. This issue can often be avoided by visiting an orthodontist early, like age seven or eight, to diagnose the likelihood of the issue and sometimes to remove the baby teeth in advance. So now you have a preview of the next chapter.

TAKEAWAYS

- ➡ How we look is very important in twenty-first-century America, as it was in previous centuries and is in other cultures all over the world.

- ➡ Studies show our self-esteem is dependent in part on our physical attractiveness. How we look affects how we feel.

- ➡ Teens are particularly susceptible to bad self-image based on their visage because other kids are unfiltered in their teasing and bullying.

- ➡ Social media magnifies these effects because it is instant, ubiquitous, and worldwide.

- ➡ Straightening teeth goes a long way toward helping teens fit in better, avoid bullying, and feel better about themselves. Even if orthodontic treatment were simply about cosmetics, it would still be extremely valuable.

- ➡ Orthodontics address a wide range of health issues that can result from malocclusions, including but not limited to gum disease, chewing and swallowing, and neck and head pain.

CHAPTER 4

"DO I NEED TO WAIT UNTIL ALL MY PERMANENT TEETH ARE IN?"

SAM WAS MY PATIENT for one day a few years ago. His mother brought him in at the age of eight or nine for the recommended checkup. Most children that age don't require orthodontic treatment, for a reason I'll get to in just a minute, but occasionally we see preteen children who desperately need intervention.

Sam was part of that minority of children who would be well served by a small amount of orthodontic treatment at an early age. When I felt around in his mouth, I could tell that his adult teeth were ready to erupt and his baby teeth did not appear close to falling out and making room.

While we are born without teeth, our lower incisors begin erupting around six months of age. The complete set of twenty baby teeth are usually in place by age three. These teeth are smaller, whiter, smoother, and more brittle than the adult teeth, as they only serve as a temporary bridge to our permanent dental set of thirty-two teeth.

Baby teeth serve several key functions besides allowing children to bite and chew. Baby teeth protect the gums that will be needed to support the permanent set of teeth from disease and decay. They aid in speech and normal facial appearance. And, critically, they serve as space holders for the permanent teeth.

At around age six, adult teeth are given the signal to push through our gums. As they put pressure upon the roots of our baby teeth, those roots begin to dissolve, causing the teeth to loosen and fall out. The adult teeth then grow into the vacated space. At least, that is the battle plan, but as the Prussian field general Helmuth Von Moltke once said, no battle plan survives contact with the enemy.

I recommend parents bring their children to us early so we can diagnose the problem before it arises.

Sometimes, the adult tooth is not slotted correctly and begins emerging in front of or, more commonly, behind the baby tooth. The root of the baby tooth remains strong, forcing the adult tooth to poke through the gum beside it. The result is a second row of teeth, sometimes called shark's teeth or fangs, depending on which teeth are involved. Occasionally, side or back teeth can even erupt through the palate or become impacted inside the palate or beneath the gum line.

The aesthetic and functional problems this causes are fairly evident. If the baby teeth remain intact, the child will have teeth randomly dispersed in their mouth, oriented in random directions. This is not healthy for any of the functions that teeth are designed for and can quickly cause damage to gums, the palate, the tongue, and other teeth.

Correcting this problem after the fact may require removing those stubborn baby teeth and applying braces to pull the offending adult teeth into the dental line. To avoid that, I recommend parents bring their children to us early so we can diagnose the problem before it arises.

Fortunately, Sam's mother heeded that advice, and we had the opportunity to recommend removal of the baby teeth to allow the adult teeth to emerge normally. Unfortunately, his mother rejected this advice and decided instead to roll the dice. If you've ever been to Las Vegas, you know that the house usually wins.

Sure enough, Sam returned to us two years later with a whole set of permanent teeth in the wrong position. At this point, his mother recognized that there was a problem that had to be resolved orthodontically. The result is that instead of allowing us to pull four baby teeth, which were going to fall out eventually anyway, and facilitate the proper growth of his permanent teeth, we instead were forced to admit him to a full orthodontic regimen that included more than the usual eighteen months of braces and retainers. This was very possibly a $5,000 mistake, not to mention the inconvenience to Sam of two years in braces.

What was so frustrating about Sam's case is that his mother avoided the most common mistake parents make about their children's teeth in the first place by bringing him to the orthodontist at a young age. My staff was perplexed why she would act so proactively on the one hand and then, having learned what a wise decision that was, refuse to follow through with very minor prophylactic treatment.

Much more commonly we see patients with shark's teeth who were never seen by an orthodontist and whose dentist didn't recognize the risk of permanent teeth emerging out of slot before the actual event. Thus my advice to all parents: bring your child to the orthodontist for one checkup around age seven so he or she can assess their mouth and head off any future issues.

During my two-year residency in orthodontics at the Medical College of Virginia, I published a paper in the *Journal of the American Dental Association* on this very subject. I discovered a way to determine whether young patients may be susceptible to having an upper canine tooth become impacted in their palate.

Identifying this problem years in advance allows us to intervene orthodontically, usually by extracting the baby teeth that stand in the way and will soon fall out. Simply extracting the baby teeth potentially prevents costly and painful surgery, and all its side effects, in those we treat.

That wasn't exactly the issue with Sam, but the result—avoiding future orthodontic issues—would have been the same if his mother had credited our expertise.

THE WAITING IS THE HARDEST PART

So back to the question that frames this chapter: Do we need to wait until our permanent teeth are in to consider braces? The answer is almost, but not quite, always.

In the vast majority of cases, when children walk through our doors for the first time at seven or eight years of age, they will walk out having endured nothing more than a phalanx of warm smiles and my hands poking around inside their mouths. Because we are dealing with baby teeth that will soon fall out, there is little point in bracing their teeth. Not only will that bracing almost certainly have no effect on the emerging adult teeth, but the braces themselves will lose their efficacy as the teeth to which they are attached loosen. The whole idea of bracing baby teeth simply to straighten them is laughable to any self-respecting orthodontist.

Before we move forward, it might be useful to provide an orthodontic glossary. I won't necessarily employ this numeric matrix of terms, but it might be useful for examination of the studies linked here.

There are three classes of bites described by dentists and orthodontists. The first one is rarely discussed because it is a normal or balanced bite. That is known as Class I.

Class II malocclusions occur when the lower teeth are positioned farther back and the upper teeth are farther forward. This may also involve the lower jaw being positioned too far back. It can create that classic "bucktooth" appearance that may lead to severe teasing or potentially may cause some long-term functional issues. I have been referring to this as an overjet or buck teeth.

Class III malocclusions describe the opposite—when the upper teeth are positioned farther back and the lower teeth jut forward. This is known as an underbite, and it usually involves some structural issue of the mandible, or lower jaw. It is less common and more complicated to resolve.

You might be shocked to discover the regularity with which children and parents enter our office demanding braces. In some instances, the child simply yearns to fit in with the crowd, as I noted in chapter 2, or to add even more to their social bona fides, be like the older kids. More often, the child's teeth look like a broken fence with pickets leaning every which way and random gaps between them. An adult set of teeth in this condition would warrant immediate treatment; it doesn't generally in children.

Most children, in most cases, adapt pretty quickly to their dental house of horrors and figure out how to eat and chew. By the time they're eight or nine, their adult teeth are starting to emerge anyway, so it won't be long before they will no longer have to endure the current state of affairs. In fact, it is rarely the children who are most adamant about getting braces too young; it is their mothers. If I may play armchair psychologist for a moment, I think this is some combination of embarrassment at their child's appearance, maternal (it's almost always the mothers) concern for their child's physical and emotional well-being, and overwrought empathy that projects their mortification and humiliation on a child who is significantly less concerned.

Karen and her ten-year-old daughter Maddy came to see us seeking some kind of resolution of Maddy's significant dental issues. She had such a serious overbite that her bottom teeth were impinging on her palate, causing pain and pushing her upper teeth even farther out. Any orthodontist can tell you that the most efficient course of treatment in a case like this is to wait a year or so. As her adult teeth grow in, the situation will be amenable to comprehensive therapy.

Orthodontics is as much about how patients feel as about how their teeth function.

I could also see that Maddy was in real discomfort and that Karen was near tears. This is a case where some tentative orthodontic intervention can address the main symptom—pain—without infringing on the child's life or costing the family an arm and a leg.

One thing I tell parents in these situations is that I don't know their child or their emotional needs after ten minutes in my exam room. Preadolescence can be a crucial age for emotional development, and a significant factor in that is appearance, as I've already discussed. If peers are abusing them because their dental and craniofacial issues are causing a distorted facial appearance, we may have to do something even if they are fine functionally. We can't always wait until the child is twelve to offer some kind of salve to their pain. Orthodontics is as much about how patients feel as about how their teeth function.

It is also about how patients' parents feel, since they are footing the bill. Parents often feel guilty about their children's physical abnormalities and emotional struggles. My staff go out of their way to remind parents that this is not their fault, that it is not evidence of bad parenting, and that what they are experiencing is not unusual. I'm afraid that doesn't often relieve their psychological pain.

For those parents who feel compelled to address their children's orthodontic issues before all the adult teeth are in, my staff and I explain the cost-benefit situation and let them make their own determination. I'm not talking about entering a child into a full regimen of braces on baby teeth but some orthodontic care to ameliorate the situation they face. We promise those parents who opt for treatment primarily to give their children a more normal life that we will discount the cost of future treatment if the child needs it once their adult teeth come in.

I gave Karen three options without comment, knowing that almost no matter how I framed them she, was going to choose the middle way. I told her that we could do nothing and let nature take its course. That was pretty clearly unacceptable to both Karen and Maddy. I offered to apply braces to some of Maddy's teeth, which would begin to change their position enough to eliminate the contact the lowers were making with the palate within a few weeks. Finally, I offered to make Maddy a retainer that covers the palate so the bottom teeth struck it rather than the roof of the mouth, silencing the pain without curing the unfortunate aesthetics of her mouth.

In effect, what I was proposing was the following: nothing; something dramatic; or something simple and stopgap; with concomitant costs. Karen, as predicted, and quite sensibly, chose the retainer. This addresses the pain but not the cosmetic issue. Maddy will have to withstand one more year of emotional vulnerability in school before she blossoms into the beauty she will eventually be.

We sometimes hear from parents who believe that early intervention of the primary teeth, though perhaps misguided, will save time and money in the long run, but sadly that is not the case. Straightening baby teeth does not confer any knowledge on the gums or adult teeth that would heighten the probability of two perfect dental rows.

Most of the clients who enter hoping they or their child will hear that braces are appropriate leave understanding that the problem might resolve itself when the permanent teeth arrive and, if it doesn't, that they can return for appropriate treatment in a couple of years. I promise them that I am not in the business of turning away customers willy-nilly; I pay the mortgage and put food on the family table by treating people who need or want orthodontic treatment, and I find that work extremely rewarding. I just don't treat people whom I can't help. I tell these mothers who are disappointed that their suffering child isn't a good candidate for braces yet but to "save your money." They can always pay me later.

THERE ARE MANY EXCEPTIONS

I treated one child who, as a baby, loved to suck on his binky upside down. The wider part of the pacifier pushed his upper back teeth outward so that they did not meet his lower back teeth, a malocclusion called a posterior crossbite. Upper and lower teeth that are out of line with each other inhibit chewing and can lead to a cascade of oral issues. In addition, using the pacifier this way, and especially beyond the age of three, can change the shape of the palate, in this case triggering a collapsed arch. Flattening of the palate narrows the airway and is a risk factor for a whole host of breathing, swallowing, and dental issues and must be corrected early in a child's life.

We do see some children present to us with oral issues arising from prolonged pacifier use and thumb sucking. By and large, there is nothing wrong with either; the sucking reflex is natural and calming for babies and children in their first few years. The experts recommend that after age four, pacifiers should be removed from children, though I don't believe any health professional has yet suggested removal of thumbs.

I blame the child's father for this child's extended binky use, because if I blamed his mother I would be in hot water with my wife. Yes, the child in question was my own third son, Zachary. Fortunately, this is one of those issues that can be tackled orthodontically early on and with ease, primarily with a palatal expander. The boy's father was obsessive about his son's compliant use of the appliance, and the issue was quickly resolved.

Another prescribed early intervention involves certain types of underbites in which the top front teeth drop in behind the bottoms and push the lower incisors, or side teeth, forward. Because the roots of the incisors are bearing constant pressure, this wears away a notch in the outside of the upper incisors, the same way the water from a flowing river alters the shape of a rock in the riverbed.

Correcting this early prevents permanent damage to the incisors.

There is some controversy in the profession about certain types of early interventions. Orthodontists disagree about whether to treat younger children with the classic overjet, or buck teeth, when caused by the lower jaw's displacement well inside the upper jaw. A University of Washington study twenty years ago found that when orthodontists were questioned in a blind study, they themselves could find no efficacy in treating cases with "mixed dentition" (i.e., when the child has both primary and permanent teeth).[9] Because of that finding, I usually decline service in such cases until the child has all their adult teeth. That said, I don't believe this is quite doctrine among clinicians and wouldn't be shocked if a new study offered contrary evidence that sparked a rush to treatments.

Studies suggest that whatever advantages arise from early treatment are erased over time by continued jaw growth. There may be some situations that are so dire that we would recommend early intervention, but there is such a thing as being too clever by half. In most of the cases with young children, we should simply let nature takes its course. Nature is responsible for the miracle that brought us to life in the first place, and it usually

These are judgment calls by a profession that learns more and improves every year. If we already knew it all, it wouldn't be called a practice.

---

9   G. J. King et al., "Orthodontists' Perceptions of the Impact of Phase 1 Treatment for Class II Malocclusion on Phase 2 Needs," *Journal of Dental Research* 78, no. 11 (November 1, 1999): 1745–1753, https://doi.org/10.1177/00220345990780111201.

finds some equilibrium over time. This has worked for me as a general guiding principle; of course, orthodontists tread where nature has hiccuped, so I'm not above trying to improve upon it. I just have a default position of leaving eight-year-olds alone unless I can be sure I can help them.

These are judgment calls by a profession that learns more and improves every year. If we already knew it all, it wouldn't be called a practice.

In the next chapter, we will look at the headgear that I mentioned and consider the advances in orthodontics in the last half century.

TAKEAWAYS

➡ It is recommended that children see an orthodontist at around the age of seven or eight for early detection of problems that may arise later.

➡ In the vast majority of cases, children that young are not ready for braces or other orthodontic intervention, primarily because their adult teeth are not in yet.

➡ Some children and their parents are desperate for braces before adolescence, mostly for aesthetic or emotional reasons. That is generally not a reasonable basis for treatment, although serious psychosocial considerations might lead to modest treatment.

➡ There are certain conditions that require early intervention. Prophylactic treatment can avoid costly and inconvenient treatment a few years later.

➡ There are some conditions that divide the orthodontic community. Some believe that early intervention would be beneficial, and others don't. These cases are a matter of controversy, but the empirical evidence suggests we should just let nature take its course.

➡ Orthodontics is science, but even within a science there is room for interpretation and reconsideration of old ideas. That is how we learn and improve.

not out in public. I don't think I have ordered headgear more than half a dozen times in my entire professional career.

Why that is can be attributed to advances in the field that make headgear unnecessary. In the days when my father practiced orthodontics, this extraoral device was prescribed in children to alter the relative position of the upper and lower jaws without anchoring the pulling force to the teeth that are constituents of that jaw. It was also used in adults or nongrowing adolescents to control the direction of force required to close a gap between teeth. Simply coaxing the two teeth toward each other over time results in each tooth moving about equally toward the middle. Headgear was employed to create an external anchor point so that more pressure could be applied to one tooth than the other, moving them together toward a point that is not equidistant between them.

For obvious reasons that are psychological and logistical rather than functional, the profession discovered simple replacements that are unobtrusive and comfortable. I know this firsthand, because before I ever applied this remedy to a patient, I tried it on myself. And by "tried it," I mean I implanted a screw into my own jawbone. When I realized that it didn't hurt at all and caused mild soreness for about a day, I was ready to begin prescribing it for patients.

That is one of the remedies: temporary implants that screw into the jawbone like drywall screws to anchor one tooth while another is moved toward the anchor tooth. We apply a dab of anesthetic gel to the surface of the gum and then insert the implant into the space between teeth.

The procedure itself is painless, and what little soreness follows is the result of the implant asserting pressure on the roots of the contiguous teeth. I felt a dull ache the next day, but it didn't infringe on my daily activities. For someone already undergoing orthodontic treatment, which involves applying constant pressure on various teeth all at once, the dull ache is probably lost among all the nerve signals being sent from the mouth anyway.

The derivation of this advance in orthodontics is both accidental and from outside the field, as are many inventions. Pavlov was not trying to prove anything about behaviorist responses in dogs; Roy Plunkett invented Teflon while experimenting with refrigerants; and Percy Spencer was tinkering with microwave weapons for the US Navy during World War II when the chocolate bar in his pocket melted—benefiting everyone's kitchen.

Dentists have long used implants to anchor prosthetic teeth, but those implants become permanently embedded in the jawbone—a process called osteointegration that is similar to the way tree roots incorporate man-made objects in their way. At some point while innovating a method of replacing missing teeth with a bridge, dentists found that the implants they were using as anchors came loose, undermining their effectiveness. Dentistry's loss was orthodontics' gain, and today temporary implants are used often.

Early in my career, I attended a seminar to learn optimal use of the implant from an orthodontist who spoke passionately about its utility and effectiveness. Both intrigued and mildly skeptical that anything works as well as its most ardent advocate promises, I returned to my office the following week and had the implant inserted in my own jaw, where it resides today. If you don't exert any force against it, it's more permanent than temporary, though of course it isn't performing any useful function. It does provide an awfully powerful case against the fears of a child or the reticence of a parent when I yank down my cheek and show how benign the implant is. Imagine how you would feel if your orthodontist promised you that drilling a screw into your mandible wasn't going to hurt—and then opened his own mouth to reveal the implant randomly sticking through his own jaw.

For most of my patients, my assurances and first-person account are sufficient, and we move ahead with the implant. What has amused me over the years is who remains petrified despite this evidence: it isn't the dainty, sixty-pound girls in frilly blouses; it's the burly line-backer types who, when finally cajoled into opening wide, wince in pain even before I have applied the device. I remember one thick-chested fourteen-year-old "boy's boy," who spent most of his free time tinkering with motorcycle engines, shaking with fear in anticipation of the procedure. I suspect his parents felt differently about it, because we inserted one on each side of his jaw to close the spaces resulting from congenitally missing teeth, saving the family thousands of dollars.

And when it was done, he sheepishly admitted that it didn't hurt.

While headgear has now been banished mostly to the dustbin of history, the implant is a useful tool but hardly the panacea its early adopters promised. I use the implant where appropriate, most often to move teeth into the space where congenitally absent permanent teeth are missing. This is most common in the lower second premolars (the wide grinders in the back) and lateral incisors (next to your front teeth).

Headgear does still have a role in orthodontics when a patient suffers from an underdeveloped maxilla (upper jaw) that causes the mandible (lower jaw) to stick beyond it in a classic underbite. The headgear can be worn overnight to pull the maxilla forward while maintaining a backward pressure on the mandible while patients sleep. That arrangement is still not optimal—you try sleeping with a catcher's mask on your face—which is one reason its use is so rare. Even Yogi Berra didn't wear his equipment to bed—as far as we know. But he did note that "you can observe a lot by watching."

ADVANCEMENTS IN THE PRACTICE OF ORTHODONTICS

The replacement of headgear with implants was a significant step forward for orthodontic patients, but it doesn't even earn a place on my Mount Rushmore of most important advances in the profession during my three-decade-plus career. The big three, in my view, are preadjusted braces, direct bonding, and clear aligners. Let's take a look at each.

(I realize that Mount Rushmore comprises four presidents and I'm listing just a Top Three of innovations, so it could be argued that implants are the fourth great advance. I would consider it a distant fourth, if it even is fourth, so perhaps this is more like the four Beatles, with implants being the Ringo Starr of the quartet.)

PREADJUSTED OR STRAIGHT-WIRE BRACES

The first advance in the Top Three is the preadjusted, or straight-wire, appliance. To understand its value, it is imperative first to understand the basic functioning of braces.

In a nutshell, braces are metal brackets attached to teeth and connected to an arch wire set by an orthodontist to pull the teeth slowly over time into the desired position. In the early days, the arrangement required the orthodontist to adjust the wire individually on every tooth to approximate the optimal tooth alignment.

Orthodontists working before 1970 had the ability to create beautiful smiles, but it was more painstaking and less predictable.

For decades until 1970, orthodontists were required to bend the wire themselves in the hope that they could account for tooth morphology and root angulation in every tooth. Perfecting the wire position was difficult and time consuming, and prone to small errors as a result.

Orthodontists working before 1970 had the ability to create beautiful smiles, but it was more painstaking and less predictable.

In 1970, the preadjusted, or straight-wire, appliance was introduced, expediting the process and producing better results for patients. The preadjusted brackets have the ideal tip, torque, angulation, and position built into each bracket, removing some of the human element from their application. Different straight-wire braces are designed for each type of malocclusion: one for underbites, another for overbites, still another for overjets, and so on, and they are optimized for average cases.

Undoubtedly, the orthodontist will nonetheless be required to adjust the wire for each individual case that is not "average," but with less adjusting, the result is almost always a clearer path to a happy smile.

DIRECT BONDING

The next great leap in orthodontics also took place in the 1970s. Until that time, brackets were welded to metal bands wrapped around each individual tooth, resulting in that quintessential railroad-track or metal-mouth look so dreaded by patients, particularly teenagers. The application of braces literally demanded that the orthodontist apply a bracket that circumnavigated each tooth. For decades before the 1970s, orthodontists bemoaned the lack of an adhesive that could bond the bracket to enamel without microscopic gaps that would allow food and bacteria to penetrate and destroy teeth. The idea for direct bonding was commonly discussed inside the profession, but its use advanced in fits and starts as bonding agents were found wanting.

By the 1980s, when I began practicing, bonding agents were formulated and perfected, and their advantages were immediately evident. From an aesthetic standpoint, attaching brackets directly to the front of teeth has transformed orthodontics. Rather than present a mouth entirely encased in metal, patients today can smile with braces, confident that the whites of their teeth remain visible.

Oral hygiene remains critical during the eighteen months or more that patients wear their braces. With wraparound brackets, brushing and flossing was compromised by the inaccessibility of much of the tooth. Bonding agents that allow no daylight between the bracket and the tooth make brushing and flossing a simpler operation, though no less imperative. Patients noncompliant with dedicated oral hygiene promote the growth of bacteria and plaque from food particles trapped in the braces. Bacteria—the same culprits that cause cavities—can create demineralization of the teeth; that is, the bacteria begin to break down the enamel and destroy the tooth.

Direct bonding also has orthodontic benefits, including the elimination of the need for posttreatment space closure between teeth. In short, direct bonding has revolutionized the practice of orthodontics during my career, making braces a more attractive option for more people.

THE CLEAR ALIGNER REVOLUTION

Imagine you went to the orthodontist in 1996 expecting to join the millions who have endured the gauntlet of metal braces and all their life-limiting implications, at least for the two years of treatment. Instead, your orthodontist proposed to provide you a series of nearly invisible mouth guards that could be removed during meals and brushing during the eighteen months it would take for them to correct your bite. No doubt that orthodontist would have been the toast of the town.

It didn't happen quite that way, but clear aligners are the third and greatest advance in orthodontics, and the most recent. Initially developed by Invisalign, there are now numerous alternatives that correct malocclusions in a less intrusive way. Simply put, Invisalign has changed the world.

(I am going to use *Invisalign* and *clear aligners* interchangeably, because although there are now others, Invisalign did invent clear aligners and were the only manufacturers of the clear aligner for many years.)

Clear aligners move teeth somewhat differently than braces and provide a plethora of benefits. For orthodontists, the major advance produced by clear aligners is 3D computer technology—computer-aided design and manufacturing—that digitally plans the exact progress of tooth movement over the course of treatment. With braces, the orthodontist has a plan for tooth alignment in his or her mind's eye that may be adjusted somewhat over the course of treatment. Invisalign instead offers more exact science that guides the progress of treatment.

For patients, clear aligners are discreet, comfortable, and removable. They don't require as much time in the orthodontist's chair enduring the application of metal, adhesive, and wire. The implications for oral health are immense, and anytime a patient wishes not to have anything in or on their mouth—their wedding, for example—the aligner can simply be removed.

I will expound in more detail in the next chapter on the Invisalign revolution, including its shortcomings, limitations, and serpentine history, and explain why many teens nonetheless prefer metal braces. Suffice it to say that clear aligners have become an important part of the orthodontic tool belt, adding another tool that is right for many jobs but not for all. It is a bit like adding a nail gun to a construction worker's tool belt: it is generally preferable to manually nailing with a hammer, but it may be difficult to fit into tight spaces and can't be used with nuance the way a hammer can in the hands of a skilled craftsman. A nail gun is the right tool for securing two pieces of wood together, but it is clearly the wrong tool for a host of other functions, like turning a screw, cutting tile, bending aluminum siding, and so on. That is why there are many pockets in a tool belt.

THE WIDE WORLD OF BRACES

As I have described, the practice of moving teeth to cure malocclusions and the oral health issues that cascade from them has advanced significantly in the past few decades. I have described the big three improvements, but many smaller innovations are being unveiled with regularity. Orthodontists now have a wide array of choices in bracing patients' teeth. For example, in the early twentieth century, orthodontic braces were fashioned in gold because it is soft and malleable. Fourteen karat and eighteen karat gold was used for wires, bands, clasps, and spurs. As you can imagine, this was extraordinarily expensive, certainly not something the masses could afford. Silver was sometimes substituted for gold because it was less expensive, but its price advantage was offset by a decrease in flexibility. Other metals were out of the question for a variety of reasons, including toxicity. Metals that are prone to leaching can poison the user.

These two metals were the most popular for braces until the 1960s, when orthodontists began using stainless steel. Steel is an alloy of iron and carbon used in a wide variety of industrial products. Adding chromium or other metals to the mixture creates stainless steel, a heat- and rust-resistant metal that is light enough for braces and will hold its shape even when rolled into a wire.

Less expensive than silver; stronger, more durable, and almost as flexible as gold; and resistant to the acids common inside a mouth, high-grade stainless steel has become the standard for traditional braces today.

THE RAINBOW WORLD OF ELASTIC BANDS

The rubber bands that surround the brackets on the front of teeth during orthodontic treatment, also known as elastic ligatures, can be a source of enjoyment in patients, particularly younger patients. The ligatures come in an ever-expanding array of colors to match a patient's mood or outfit, show solidarity for a favorite team, or reflect an upcoming event or holiday. I mentioned during the discussion of clear aligners that some teens prefer traditional braces despite the various advantages of Invisalign: the color wheel is the primary reason for that. Since they are going to have their teeth straightened anyway, some teenagers—not a few—rejoice at the prospect of joining the metal-mouth club and personalizing their look. Bands come in the full Pantone color swatch of choices; if you can conjure it in your head, the color is available. Forget about bright hues of red, orange, pink, purple, green and blue; those are for people who lack imagination. My patients choose from among mauve, taupe, avocado, nectarine, razzmatazz, coquelicot (a red-tinted orange), smaragdine (an emeraldy green) and mikado (a dark yellow). For the most daring, even those are too tame: they dare to wear glittery silver and gold. It doesn't stop there; they can mix and match, too, so during late June and early July we prepare for an onslaught of requests for red, white, and blue. What a time to be a teen!

It is not unusual in my practice for a young patient to arrive for their appointment excited about the color they have chosen for this month's bands. The bands are disposable in the first place, so these budding artists have the joyous opportunity to swap out colors every time they come in for an adjustment.

CLEAR OR TOOTH-COLORED CERAMIC BRACES

Another alternative that appeals to a lot of people, particularly adults, is clear porcelain or plastic braces. With advances in the chemistry of polymers, these inorganic braces are now stronger than ever and can be used in place of stainless steel. They work the same way and are almost invisible on teeth (but not quite!). They also come in different colors, so some users can customize the color of their braces to the color of their teeth.

Ceramic braces have their drawbacks. They are bulkier and more of a challenge to apply. Because they are weaker and more brittle than stainless steel, they have been found to break twice as often. They take longer to align teeth and require more bracket adjustments and a more delicate touch by the orthodontist. Consequently, treatment with ceramic braces generally takes longer than with metal.

I use ceramic braces regularly—whenever patients request them. One recent example really brings home their value. Laura is a local journalist who had spent her entire career in print but was transitioning to video and was concerned about how braces would look on the screen. I told her she was a prime candidate for Invisalign, with her minor crossbite, but she had heard stories from friends who complained about difficulty with speech that is sometimes associated with aligners. In my experience, this difficulty lasts about fifteen minutes until the patient adapts to having plastic over their teeth, but Laura was operating with an understandable abundance of caution, so she asked instead for ceramic braces. (She also mentioned her conviction that she lacked the discipline to keep the aligners in her mouth because she is constantly snacking, which requires their removal. I've learned to trust patients who assert their lack of self-control.)

Laura's attractiveness is no doubt an asset in her new job, so it was incumbent upon both of us to get this right. At that moment of truth when I attached her new porcelain braces, she looked at me and said, "Yeah, that's what I mean." Unless the camera zooms in unusually tight on her face, the viewer won't even know she has braces on.

Some patients are not candidates for ceramic braces. They tend to inflame gums and stain teeth if oral hygiene is not meticulously maintained. Users are encouraged to avoid smoking, drinking much besides water, and limiting the amount of staining food they consume, like tomatoes, ketchup, and mustard. Patients with ceramic braces are also warned against brushing with whitening toothpaste unless they want two-tone teeth. The whitening agents can only lighten the exposed segment of the teeth, not the part under the brackets. (There are bleaching kits available for use with braces that avoid this problem.) I discourage parents of young teens who don't have good intrinsic motivation to brush and floss from making this choice.

As I've mentioned before, kids frequently want their braces as a membership card into the club of cool kids. They rock color-popping rubber bands, show off their metal, and know that straight teeth are on their way. It's rare that youngsters request ceramic braces, which hides their badge of honor. An adolescent girl came to me recently prepared for braces, when her mother pushed her to get ceramics so they wouldn't be so noticeable. She reluctantly agreed, and it appeared she had been defeated. Well. As any parent reading this knows, children generally get what they want if they are bound and determined. By adding splashes of color in the elastic bands, the daughter reclaimed her individuality, utterly defeating the ceramic aesthetic. Final score: Daughter—1, Mom—0.

LINGUAL BRACES STAY OUT OF THE WAY

Lingual braces are a fancy way of describing traditional braces that are applied to the back of the teeth instead of the front. The cosmetic advantage of this process is obvious because with braces on the inside of the mouth, they are not ordinarily apparent. Attaching braces inside the mouth is a complicating factor as the orthodontist must reach his or her hand inside the mouth and employ their usual expertise upside down and backward. That isn't in and of itself a problem; anyone with a dental degree has perfected the art of working with mirrors inside the mouth.

But it does significantly lengthen the time needed to attach lingual braces and hike the cost. Because of their difficulty with applying, many orthodontists simply don't bother with lingual braces, opting instead for ceramic braces or clear aligners when cosmetic issues are paramount.

For those who do, lingual braces have been found to produce the same results as traditional braces once affixed. Patients also have less trouble brushing their teeth and maintaining oral hygiene on the lip and cheek surface of the teeth. I use lingual braces when patients demand them, but there are better alternatives, and I don't recommend them. I've probably done a dozen in my thirty years of practice.

Lingual braces have a few other shortcomings, the worst being that they create a lisp in the user. When speaking, the tongue makes contact with the back of teeth for the production of certain sounds, like *t, d, j, l, z,* and, most significantly, *s.* Lingual braces interfere with that process. A study in the *Dental Research Journal* found that the aesthetic advantage of lingual braces is "eclipsed by the drawback that the bracket placement on the lingual surface entails a substantial, albeit temporary, change in the morphology of the lingual tooth surface due to the brackets and thus of the second articulation zone."[10] These studies found that patients acclimated to the appliance in a month or two.

Indeed, lingual braces are often simply more uncomfortable than traditional braces. It takes patients more time to get accustomed to having metal inside their mouths than outside. The inside of the mouth exposes more soft tissue to the braces; in fact, tongue irritation, soreness, and pain are the most common complaints of patients with this appliance. Topical pain relief usually dulls the discomfort and allows time for patients to adapt. Manufacturers are now producing smaller and smoother lingual brackets to combat that issue. Even so, this option takes longer and costs more than traditional braces, so whatever discomfort is involved will affect the patient for longer.

Lingual braces are not indicated for patients with deep overbites. They tend to pop off more frequently, reducing their effectiveness and extending the period of treatment. Nor are they recommended for patients with bruxism—excessive teeth grinding—as they interfere with biting and chewing. Individuals who play brass or wind instruments may find that lingual braces present a difficult adjustment.

PASSIVE SELF-LIGATING BRACES

Self-ligating braces are a useful innovation. The arch wire runs through a metal door on the brace on each tooth that holds it inside the bracket, replacing the elastic ligatures found in more conventional braces. Proponents of the various self-ligating systems argue that they

---

10   Ambesh Kumar Rai et al., "Comparison of Speech Performance in Labial and Lingual Orthodontic Patients: A Prospective Study," *Dental Research Journal* 11, no. 6 (November-December 2014): 663–675, https://www.ncbi.nlm.nih.gov/pmc/articles/PMC4275635/.

take less time to adjust at the adjustment appointments because there is no need to attach rubber bands and that the movement of the wire is smoother.

Orthodontists who believe in self-ligating braces tend to use them exclusively and become adept at their use.

I have utilized self-ligating braces in the past but have largely discontinued their use for the most prosaic of reasons: kids still want the customizable elastic bands. Applying the bands defeats the purpose of self-ligating braces, leaving us with a bracing system that is significantly more expensive. As for any functional benefits, I never witnessed them and have not seen any empirical data supporting claims of superiority.

COMPUTERIZED TREATMENT SYSTEMS SAVE TIME AND ADD PERFECTION

One last innovation I'll mention is one that patients don't appreciate the way practitioners do because it is behind the scenes. I've mentioned how orthodontists during the twentieth century estimated the track teeth would take to arrive in their desired position. Technology has helped us eliminate a significant amount of approximation and provided more precise experiences. Don't get me wrong: robots haven't replaced orthodontists, and I doubt they ever will, but they have allowed professionals like me to apply our creative and artistic skill to a highly engineered process.

One example of this is the Insignia treatment system that we use in our practice. Insignia employs scanning software to take a digital impression of the teeth and jaws, ensuring the production of a customized orthodontic appliance. Insignia software is used to design the optimal plan for each patient, and robotics determine the precise placement of wires and brackets.

We employ an indirect bonding procedure with Insignia, which allows us to apply the brackets onto a mold of the patient's teeth. This saves the patient time in the orthodontist's chair because the position of each bracket is predetermined and can be applied all at once. The result of this process is a more exact fit, a more comfortable experience for the patient, and the most beautiful smile possible in the end.

The benefits of innovation in the profession have rippled out to patients of every type. Braces today are easier to apply, more comfortable to wear, more aesthetically pleasing, and custom fit so they work faster and more perfectly. In the next chapter, we're going to discuss the one giant leap for orthodontic-kind—the clear aligner—and explore all the misconceptions about it.

TAKEAWAYS

➡ Cumbersome and unsightly headgear is rarely used anymore, replaced by, among other things, temporary mini-screws that are painlessly implanted in the jawbone.

➡ Where the face-bow headgear is necessary, usually to hold the upper jaw back, it is employed at night. You will almost never see anyone walking around with this contraption during business hours.

➡ The three great advances in orthodontics during the last forty years are, in my opinion, the preadjusted or straight-wire braces, direct bonding of the brackets to teeth, and the Invisalign clear aligner.

➡ Preadjusted braces take educated guesswork out of the process by putting into orthodontists' hands bracing systems conforming to the various kinds of misalignments they are correcting.

➡ Direct bonding allows orthodontists to bond the brackets directly onto the front of the teeth rather than wrap the metal around each individual tooth. This is more comfortable, faster, and eliminates the bulky metal-mouth look.

➡ Invisalign is more than an innovation; it is a revolution. Instead of requiring patients to wear permanent metal braces, clear aligners move teeth equally well, can be removed for meals and emergencies, and are nearly invisible.

➡ There have been many more small steps forward, including but not limited to stainless steel braces, ceramic braces, lingual braces, self-ligating brackets, computerized diagnostics, and production of colored bands, all of which have their benefits and drawbacks—except colored bands, which are just plain cool.

CHAPTER 6

"INVISALIGN / CLEAR ALIGNERS ARE FOR ADULTS ONLY"

ZIA CHISHTI WAS BORN in the United States but grew up in Pakistan, the son of an American father and a Pakistani mother. He moved back to the States to matriculate at Columbia University and earn a BA in computer science and economics. After working as an investment banker, he attended Stanford University for his MBA.

Around this time, the late 1990s, Chishti was undergoing orthodontic treatment. He found it uncomfortable, even painful, and wondered whether there might be a better way. At the end of treatment, his doctor fitted him with a clear plastic retainer and directed him to wear it vigilantly to maintain the correction of his bite.

The common conception of breakthrough inventions is that a light bulb goes off in the inventor's head, they yell, "Eureka!" and they present to the world their invention to immediate acclaim. The truth is considerably less exciting.

Chishti repeatedly lost his retainer and, in the time it took to return to the orthodontist and get fitted with a new one, noticed his teeth shifted out of alignment. When he reinserted the new retainer, his teeth returned to their optimal position.

That got him thinking. If the retainer could move his teeth at the end of the process, a series of retainers could move teeth during the entire process and avoid the need for cumbersome braces and all the issues that ripple out from their use. Enlisting help from friends and Stanford graduate students, he set about to create 3D computer models of the retainers. Using CAD/CAM software programs and the cutting-edge 3D printing technology available at Stanford, they developed digital images and converted them into clear plastic aligners. The program they developed could model a patient's current bite and design the retainers that the patient would need to achieve the attractive, functional bite they desired.

In 1997, Chishti and three partners formed Align Technology and, in pure Silicon Valley fashion, worked out of a garage to test their invention, reduce its cost, improve its function, raise capital, and begin marketing their clear plastic aligners to orthodontists.

Angel investors jumped on board, but orthodontists did not. The inventors had no dental or orthodontic training. They were not connected to the orthodontic community in any way. They were challenging a century of orthodoxy and had no empirical data or case studies supporting their claims that a series of plastic trays could replicate the force that wires and brackets produced to move teeth. To be fair, employing a new orthodontic system without any proof of concept puts patients at risk.

Invisalign began marketing its alternative to metal braces directly to consumers and, by 2001, had created a grassroots demand for the product, with 175,000 people swearing by the new treatment system. With more evidence of the efficacy of Invisalign, more orthodontists signed on, and Invisalign began replacing traditional braces in adults.

Because Chishti was an adult orthodontic patient, he originally designed his treatment system for adults and not children. Perhaps the major drawback of clear aligners is also one of their primary benefits—they can be removed. Invisalign marketed its system entirely for adult patients in the early years, assuming that children would be less responsible about returning the tray onto their teeth.

The Invisalign system has evolved over time and has for the last few years eliminated the need for traditional bracing at the end of treatment.

I was an early adopter of Invisalign but, I must admit, not an early convert. I used clear aligners in the early 2000s before they had really gained traction in the orthodontic community, but I was skeptical about their use. At that time, the Invisalign system was not sufficiently refined to achieve good finishes; it could only accomplish about 80 percent of the treatment. Even when I was using Invisalign, it was a hybrid treatment plan that ended with braces. After a while I began to question why I bothered with Invisalign in the first place if I had to put my patients in metal braces eventually, and my use of the clear aligners waned.

Fortunately, the Invisalign system has evolved over time and has for the last few years eliminated the need for traditional bracing at the end of treatment. In fact, Invisalign is indicated for virtually any kind of malocclusion that can be remedied with braces. Remember Teddy from chapter 3? His teeth were a cornucopia of malocclusions, and we are perfecting his smile with a series of Invisalign trays. As a result, I employ Invisalign for most of my adult patients and many of my child patients.

THE EVOLUTION OF INVISALIGN

Invisalign has just two decades of use under its belt, and in that time the system has advanced dramatically. In its first and second iterations, manufacturing the aligner was messy, time consuming, and required a third party whose involvement slowed the process. Today it is clean, quick, in-house, and more precise.

At the start of the Invisalign revolution, the orthodontist instructed the patient to bite into a goopy substance to create a mold of the teeth. The orthodontist then created a stone model from the impression and generally had the aligners fabricated in a lab from that. This process was repeated two or three more times during the process. The common response by patients to this process was … "Yuck!"

Patient reactions to the alginate impression—the goo—was so negative that Invisalign switched to a PVS impression, which is more like rubber cement. Though less messy than alginate, it did require that the impression be mailed to a lab that could scan it into a digital mold and then create a digital tooth manipulation plan. Once approved by the orthodontist, the lab would create 3D print models from which to fabricate the aligners and then mail them back. This was a dramatic improvement in every way but temporal; that is, it wasted a lot of time.

Today, the system is streamlined considerably for the benefit of the patient and the orthodontist. Now that every orthodontist can own a scanner and some digital 3D manipulation tools, the treatment plan can be developed in a day or two and the scans can be uploaded to Invisalign for significantly expedited aligner production.

BENEFITS OF INVISALIGN

If you were to ask my patients why they prefer clear aligners to traditional metal braces, they would almost universally identify the cosmetic advantages and ease of use. Because clear aligners are hardly noticeable, adults particularly appreciate the ability to develop a beautiful smile without feeling like outcasts in the process. In addition, because they are removable, like a mouth guard used for sports, patients can take them out when they eat, avoiding the complication of food getting stuck in metal braces. Invisalign patients face

Invisalign works faster in many cases than traditional braces because the movement of teeth is continuous and predictable.

no restrictions on eating hard foods that can break metal braces, as long as they brush and floss regularly. But everyone should be brushing and flossing regularly anyway.

Clear aligners are also more comfortable than braces because there are no metal parts rubbing against gums, tongue, or lips. Because they have no wires and rubber bands that can break, wearing clear aligners means fewer unscheduled trips to the orthodontist for repairs. With Invisalign, no patient has ever called on Christmas Eve with broken braces or a wire sticking into their cheek that necessitated an urgent visit to my office.

These are what patients would identify as the advantages of clear aligners.

If you ask an orthodontist, the primary benefit of Invisalign is the computer technology that creates a clear, precise treatment plan at the beginning of the process. Using artificial intelligence that learns from the millions of cases now in its database, Invisalign has improved the accuracy of its software. Its clear aligners do every bit as good a job of moving teeth as traditional braces—in most cases.

Invisalign works faster in many cases than traditional braces because the movement of teeth is continuous and predictable. The orthodontist knows in advance how and how much teeth will move. The next step is predetermined and simply requires switching trays. With metal braces, it is more challenging to titrate movement precisely; consequently, the orthodontist must see the patient frequently to review the movement of teeth and adjust the plan accordingly. Patients with braces return to the orthodontist every six weeks on average compared to every two months with Invisalign. For patients who live far away, we even conduct periodic virtual consultations and invite them to wait three months before returning.

BUILDING CONFIDENCE WITH INVISALIGN

Ron is a financial advisor for a major national financial services company. A lot of people around town know him, which is important in his job.

Financial advising, like a lot of things in life, is all about relationships. People need to know Ron and feel comfortable with him, his expertise, his ability, and his integrity before they are going to give him their life savings to invest. His livelihood is literally predicated on making a good impression on everyone he meets, because everyone is a potential client. As I documented before, a large part of what forms people's impressions of us is based on how we look.

Ron was not feeling confident about that.

He came to our office seeking a solution to his off-kilter smile. His mouth was crowded with teeth, pushing the front two into a crossover position. Ron was uncomfortable with his smile and even covered his mouth when he felt one coming on. Fixing his smile was not just aesthetic for him; it was an investment in his business.

If Ron had come to us in 2010, we would have recommended some tooth extractions to accommodate traditional bracing and many months of braces on his teeth. Invisalign was not routine in tooth extraction cases because of the way the aligner tray works on gaps in teeth. This would have been a problem for Ron. A professional in his thirties, Ron was not about to walk around with brackets and wires on his teeth like some teenybopper. That would have been death for his business and deeper embarrassment for him emotionally.

Before I go on with Ron's story, let me just say that there is nothing inevitable about feeling this way. Adults are increasingly seeking smile solutions as the process of correcting bad teeth gets easier, less uncomfortable, and relatively less expensive. Orthodontic treatment has not changed much in price over the last decade or two, making it more affordable every year. While some adults, like Ron, are mortified about the prospect of wearing braces, others find it fun—a conversation starter, even. It all depends on your frame of mind. Ron's frame of mind was not nearly as sanguine about metal braces.

The good news for him is that Invisalign has come a long way and can now be used in tooth extraction cases. We provided a full course of treatment with clear aligners that his clients could hardly notice and corrected the crowding and the crossbite. Today Ron projects a level of confidence he didn't exhibit before, business is booming, and we are now treating one of his children. It is a story with a happy ending made possible by the continuing evolution and improvement of Invisalign.

SO, CAN CHILDREN USE INVISALIGN?

One improvement that Invisalign never had to make was to adapt its treatment system to children. That clear aligners were marketed exclusively to adults at the turn of the century was simply a business decision, not the result of any clinical barrier to their use.

It may have been a result of Chishti's personal experience as an adult seeking orthodontic treatment. More likely it was a proactive determination on the part of the company that children could not be responsible enough to return their aligners to their mouths after meals. Noncompliance may be the single most significant inhibiting factor in the use of Invisalign.

I will give you an example of how that might work, but you will be surprised to discover that it involves an adult, not a child. In fact, in my experience, children are more compliant than adults, not less.

I had a patient whose name I won't use because she probably does not want the world to know that she didn't have the discipline to use Invisalign when twelve-year-old boys do.

Although patients may eat and drink what they like when they remove their aligners, they may not eat or drink anything other than water with the aligners in. Anyone addicted to consuming some food or drink—coffee, soda, bubble gum—must either kick the habit or wear braces. This woman came to us saying she had a six-a-day diet cola habit from which she wanted to break free. As long as she was having her bite fixed, she thought, she might as well get Invisalign and force herself into a cold turkey situation.

The bad news is she didn't have the willpower to keep the aligner in and eschew the drink. The good news is she was so hopelessly addicted that it became apparent within two weeks. On her first visit after being fit with the aligner, she surrendered to the addiction and directed me to install braces. We have never had that situation with a child.

Just to be safe, Invisalign has created products specifically designed for the nanosecond attention span of today's kids. In 2017 they released Invisalign Teens with features that accommodate growing teeth, keep track of the aligners' use, and offer free replacements if they are lost. I particularly like the way the aligners "tattle" on patients who don't wear them enough. A dot on the Invisalign Teen aligners changes color the more they are worn, so children who take them out and fail to replace them in their mouths are outed by the aligners themselves. Of course, this workaround is premised on the compliance of the parents, who must enforce the aligners' use. Presumably, because they are paying for orthodontic treatment, they are incentivized to exert pressure on their children to take responsibility for their aligners. It is not a fail-safe system, but there is no such thing as perfection when working with humans.

Of course, with children, it is something of a self-selected sample. We grill parents about their children before embarking on an Invisalign treatment plan. We ask if the child gets his or her homework done on time without prodding. We ask if they are always losing things, if they must be reminded to walk the dog or practice their musical instrument. We ask if they are constantly losing their glasses or their phone. For children who don't appear to be responsible and intrinsically motivated, we strongly encourage parents to opt for traditional braces. It is all the same to me and my staff: we charge the same for either.

The point is, we are weeding out the children apt to fail at compliance with Invisalign. That has helped us achieve a 95 percent compliance rate with the system. But it is worth pointing out that conventional braces require a level of compliance as well. Patients must be more vigilant about brushing and flossing. They must wear the rubber bands in many cases, or the braces won't work. Often we find that, once we have straightened their smile but before we have corrected their bite, some children with braces will become satisfied and lose interest in maintaining compliance.

It is true that patients can't take their braces off, but they can undermine the process if they are irresponsible. What we find, whether patients are in conventional braces or clear aligners, is that patients who want to correct their bite and beautify their smile are going to demonstrate the modicum of discipline required to succeed whether they are thirteen or thirty-one.

Still, if a parent is skeptical, Invisalign offers incentives to offset any risk involved. The company will guarantee that the child will love their aligner and comply with instructions to wear it twenty-two hours daily. If it becomes apparent anytime in the first six months that the child is unable to comply, Invisalign will pay to defray the cost of switching to conventional braces.

WHAT CAN'T INVISALIGN DO?

Invisalign and other clear aligners do have some minor limitations. One example that the company has attempted to address, though not to my satisfaction, is the issue of impacted teeth. A plastic tray fitted over teeth is incapable of extruding a tooth through the gum into position.

There is a workaround: inserting a glob of glue into the aligner and attaching it to a spring that pulls the tooth out when the aligner is worn. Technically this can work, but it requires the patient to attach an elastic band into the aligner every time it is removed and replaced. The chances of most patients applying such painstaking devotion to the issue are somewhere between slim and none, and Slim is saddling up to ride out of town. I have always operated on the premise that ease of use facilitates compliance; as such, if employing Invisalign is going to burden the patient, we might as well opt for one of the many options among braces.

The inefficiency of using clear aligners with surgical orthodontics—that is, when the jaw is so far out of alignment that it requires surgery to be repositioned—has also driven orthodontists into the arms of more conventional braces. In these cases, I sometimes begin the treatment with braces and, after surgery and recovery, finish the process with clear aligners.

That is a small minority of cases, leaving Invisalign as an option for most patients. As I mentioned, once upon a time clear aligners could not be employed in cases involving extractions of teeth. They also were not prescribed for extreme overbites and underbites. Generally speaking, Invisalign was not an option in cases where the relative position of the jaws—the mandible and maxilla—had to be altered. Then the company unveiled its mandibular advancement that uses wings on the side of the appliance to push the mandible forward.

In early 2020, a pair of brothers, aged fourteen and twelve, came to see us, and it was immediately clear that they were timid and anxious, one worse than the other. Colin, the younger brother, seemed to absorb the fear his older brother Mason was modeling, so the two of them quaked at the prospect of getting braces. I don't know what horror stories they had heard, but they evidently took them to heart and likely had embellished them by the time their limbic system kicked in.

Both boys needed their mandibles pulled forward to align their teeth and correct a serious overjet, or buck teeth. As recently as 2019, this would have precluded the use of Invisalign and required the very braces that shivered the duo's timbers. When I announced to them that they were in luck because Invisalign had conquered this issue with the introduction of wings, the pair were greatly relieved. In fact, this was my first foray with the wings, but they worked like a charm, and both boys made good progress. Because appointments in the case of Invisalign treatments are generally little more than a checkup, they tend to be short and nonthreatening. In the majority of cases, when everything is tracking correctly, I hand them a new series of aligners and send them on their way.

The combination of the aligners and quick checkups has served to ratchet down their discomfort level. It is rewarding to know that two cases appearing inauspicious at the outset are going to end with everyone living happily ever after.

I have mentioned on a couple of occasions how easy Invisalign and other clear aligners are for orthodontists to work with and for patients to use. You might be thinking that anyone with a scanner, some computer software, and a 3D printer could pop out these aligners and simply send them to patients with written instructions for a fraction of the cost. In fact, several companies are doing just that, much to the detriment of patients. In the next chapter, we're going to explore this new phenomenon and honestly consider whether I have legitimate concerns or just turf-protection instincts.

TAKEAWAYS

→ The Invisalign revolution was sparked not by an orthodontist but by someone with computer and business expertise who thought there must be a better way to move teeth after experiencing orthodontic treatment.

→ Invisalign was not well received at the start, in part because its inventor had no credibility with orthodontists and in part because it had many shortcomings in the early days.

→ Although Invisalign invented the clear aligner, there are now numerous other companies producing their own clear aligner systems, providing competition, sparking innovation, and keeping costs low.

→ The primary innovation offered by Invisalign is the computer-aided treatment planning in which the full complement of aligners is 3D printed at the start.

→ The primary innovation that most patients see is the cosmetic advantage of invisible bracing and the ability to remove the aligners to eat and brush teeth.

→ Over the years, Invisalign has introduced advances to allow aligner use for a wider variety of malocclusions. There are still a handful of orthodontic issues that preclude the use of Invisalign or render it less effective, but they are fewer and farther between than ever.

→ In the late 1990s and early 2000s, Invisalign could only accomplish about 80 percent of the job, but today it works just as well, faster, than conventional braces.

➡ Invisalign was originally marketed only to adults, perhaps because the company believed that teens would fail to keep the aligners in their mouths. In fact, the aligners work equally well for people of all ages, and kids have turned out to be more compliant with the protocols than adults.

➡ Just to be safe, Invisalign offers a guarantee to parents that if their child's inability to wear the appliance forces a restart with conventional braces, Invisalign will cover the cost of starting over.

CHAPTER 7

"WHAT'S THE DEAL WITH DIY ORTHODONTICS?"

I'LL NEVER FORGET the first time it happened, because my retrospective mental image of myself is of a man in a white coat, dental tools in hand, with his jaw scraping across the floor in mute astonishment. I had heard about these smile-by-mail programs and wrote them off in my mind as such a transparently bad idea, such a ridiculous health gamble, that no one in their right mind would even be tempted. I never considered that any significant number of people would think that they didn't need an orthodontist, or any medical professional at all, to engage in the highly complex science and art of moving teeth that emanate from their jawbones that are attached to their skull and can affect literally every bodily system. It seemed to me that the public would understand that this was akin to playing Russian roulette, but with three bullets chambered.

Yet in my own orthodontic chair sat a lovely midtwenties woman with a crowded mouth who undoubtedly could benefit from orthodontic care. I won't name her or offer any details of her life, because I don't want to embarrass her. Besides, she was only the first.

She didn't mention anything at first, but when I looked around in her mouth, I could see that something was amiss. While her teeth were a bit of a jumble, it appeared there had been some desultory effort to realign them, however halting. It looked as if someone had made an incompetent attempt to align only her front teeth and the treatment had started, achieved poor results, and ceased at an early stage. I asked her whether she had sought treatment previously, and only then did she admit sheepishly that she had taken an $1,800 gamble on one of those direct order teeth-straightening programs. I said nothing judgmental, but I can't vouch for my face, which must have conveyed my state of bewilderment. Only later, after more cases like this walked through our door, did I realize that this late-night TV advertising gimmick was actually catching on.

These DIY orthodontic marketers are capitalizing on the Invisalign revolution—though they are using an Invisalign knock-off system—that employs digital technology to craft customized clear aligners that require relatively little manipulation by the orthodontist. Even with an orthodontist, the key to the success of Invisalign is the patients themselves and their ability to wear the aligners as directed for twenty-two hours every day.

They are also narrowly focusing their marketing on simply straightening front teeth for a nice smile, not promising to treat malocclusions, bite issues, jaw positioning, pain, or anything else. Many of them caution that their services are only designed for minor corrections. Their work is simply a cosmetic facade. The rest of a customer's teeth don't even have to exist for them to claim they delivered on their promise. This in and of itself is not a complaint: if all someone wants is a nicer smile, they should be able to get that and not pay for any other treatment. I regularly treat patients who decline the full orthodontic regimen simply to improve their smile. The difference is that they are being treated personally by an orthodontist who can, among other things, explain to them the possible ramifications of shifting only front teeth, and the possible issues they may want to consider addressing in the rest of their mouth.

As I probed her mouth, I began inquiring into the course of the "treatment" she had received and what she thought went wrong. Back in those days, these direct mail operations required customers to bite down on goop and create their own bite mold, which they sent to the company as the foundation for treatment. What she and many others found is that patients are not generally adept at dentistry—imagine that—and their molds were poor blueprints for treatment. This is a challenge for trained dental professionals; the notion that ordinary untrained individuals were going to succeed at creating a usable mold was a pipe dream. Every dentist and orthodontist on planet Earth could have predicted poor results. More recently these companies have established scan centers where customers can go to get their teeth scanned. Where I live, an hour from Salt Lake City, customers would likely have to drive an hour and a half or more round trip for the scan. I'm not aware of any of these places convenient to people here.

Besides getting off to a bad start, she told me that once the aligners arrived, she was on her own. She received no guidance, she said, and never knew whether she was using them correctly. She said they never really fit from the first aligner on, but she had no way of knowing whether she was wearing them wrong or making some mistake in their use. As you might imagine, the problem cascaded from aligner to aligner, and as her teeth were not moving as predicted, the aligners became more ill fitting. One of the keys to patient compliance is a positive feedback loop; that is, the patient can see some progress, so they continue to follow the protocols, so they see more progress, so they stay with it, and so on. This woman not only wasn't in a positive feedback loop, she was in just the opposite—a negative feedback loop. It led her to finally give up on what was clearly not working, and she was out nearly $2,000.

The good news for her was that I could help her; in fact, Invisalign was tailor made for her issues. However, she was so soured on clear aligners that I knew she would decline that option, and she chose instead to get conventional braces, which worked just as they are supposed to in the hands of a trained professional, and she is now a lovely young woman with a beautiful smile.

Every orthodontist I know can recount similar experiences with people who tried the low-cost DIY orthodontics and instead cost themselves two grand for nothing except another year or two with misaligned teeth.

Ultimately, they found themselves in an orthodontist's chair receiving the treatment they actually needed from a medical professional and his or her trained staff.

What underlies this industry of remote tooth straightening is the notion that you don't need an educated dental professional to help you with oral issues, that straightening teeth is simply cosmetic—consequently, a computer can achieve the same results. That orthodontists spent four years in dental school, then clinical training, then two or three years of orthodontic training, earned a doctorate and various certifications, yet have no knowledge or expertise of value. Some computer technician on the other side of the country—or perhaps the world—can customize your clear aligners for you, because it is really just a series of unrelated tasks, like taking out the garbage or assembling a jigsaw puzzle.

This, of course, is absurd. The nation's ten thousand orthodontists didn't go to dental and orthodontic school and spend years honing their skills for no reason. Our work is integrative and requires a series of professional judgments. Every part of the human body is connected, so pathologies with the oral cavity can cause illness, injury, pain, and suffering elsewhere in the body. Just as one simple example that should be familiar to everyone, recent research has demonstrated that there is a link between gum disease and heart disease. People diagnosed with gingivitis or other periodontal disease are at increased risk of heart disease. The Mayo Clinic calls oral health "a window to your overall health."

AREN'T YOU GOING TO EXAMINE ME?

Here is one simple example of how DIY orthodontics steers you wrong, perhaps dangerously wrong. When a patient comes to my practice for treatment, the first thing we do is take an x-ray of their mouth. This is mostly precautionary to avoid beginning orthodontic treatment on a patient with invisible underlying issues. Recently, we treated a man whose initial x-ray revealed a dark area around the roots of the teeth in the mandible—the lower jaw. It is often dark back there, so we kept an eye on it and took another x-ray a couple of months later, which revealed the dark spot growing. We immediately halted treatment and sent him to an oral surgeon who removed and biopsied the lesion. Fortunately, it was benign, but even then, it would have continued growing and very likely consumed the roots of the teeth around it, causing several teeth to fall out and undermining our orthodontic treatment. Of course, had the lesion been cancerous, our intervention might have saved his life.

Order-by-mail aligners skip the physical exam as well. Can you imagine having any medical procedure without a doctor examining you first? You can't even give blood at the Red Cross without having your pulse, temperature, and blood pressure taken. When a patient walks into almost any orthodontist's office, the orthodontist will examine them for gum disease, bone loss, and other issues that might require treatment and could interfere with orthodontic work. Because they aren't doing a physical exam, the mail-order folks don't know if they are putting clear aligners on a customer with periodontal disease whose teeth are going to fall out after they are straightened.

These mail-order enterprises do not do physical exams or take x-rays because most physical exams and x-rays are normal, so they are not cost effective. Physical exams and x-rays are good for patients, though. These operations are failing Orthodontics 101 and elevating cost control above the health of their patients. What would you expect from a business that never meets you or gets to know you?

Perhaps you think it's a good wager even if it doesn't work out occasionally. You spend $2,000 or so, and if you don't achieve a good result, no harm done—you can always go to an orthodontist. If you like the results, you saved a few bucks on the full orthodontic treatment. The problem with that logic is twofold:

Their results are dismal.

You're not actually saving any money.

THE RESULTS ARE DISMAL

The second reason is the big one, so let's start with the first: their results are dismal. I decided to begin a search of reviews of these services, and the very first compilation I found included 138 reviews.[11] Of that number, just fifty people definitively said the service was worth the cost. That is just a 36 percent satisfaction rate. Your odds are one in three that you will look back on your smile-by-mail scheme and think, "Boy, am I smart for saving money." (The website cites a 57 percent satisfaction rate because it discounts all the "not sure" answers. You know what the "not sure" rate is in my practice? Roughly zero. In fact, dissatisfaction in our work is so rare that we solicit criticism so that we can learn and improve our practice. Imagine an orthodontist soliciting criticisms when two-thirds of their customers have some complaint and nearly half know for sure that they regretted engaging their services. The practice would be spending all day fielding complaints. An orthodontist with twice their satisfaction rate—72 percent—is likely incompetent and would be out of business in two years.)

In other words, the payoff on the bet is poor. And that isn't even the worst news for DIY orthodontics.

THERE ARE NO COST SAVINGS

Here is the real irony in all this: if all you want to accomplish is to straighten your front teeth for a nice smile and nothing more, that is a service my practice provides and always has. We offer you personalized orthodontic services—not mail-order aligners—under the care of an orthodontist and his trained staff, checking on

Simply straightening front teeth requires five to ten aligners, rather than a couple of dozen, and takes much less time.

---

11   "SmileDirectClub Reviews," RealSelf, accessed December 2020, https://www.realself.com/reviews/smiledirectclub.

you along the way, making adjustments as necessary, and standing ready to provide guidance anytime you need it. Here is the kicker: the cost of that limited service is and always has been about the same as what the DIY teeth straighteners charge. Simply straightening front teeth requires five to ten aligners, rather than a couple of dozen, and takes much less time.

People who make the mistake of sending away for aligners not only don't get good results; they aren't saving any money. Isn't that the whole point of these operations? Avoiding all that orthodontic work that takes time and money when all you want is a proper smile? These operations offer very limited services and do not provide significant savings but do have significantly worse outcomes that might require that you see an orthodontist anyway and spend that money all over again. Does that still sound like a good wager?

Let me pause here and address the elephant in the room: I am an orthodontist. It is to be expected that I am going to oppose an industry disruptor that devalues my expertise and promises to deliver more or less the same service I do at what it claims is greatly reduced cost. You might think I'm just trying to protect my turf. That would be understandable.

One could view these mail-order outfits as the next Uber, Zoom, Zappos, and so on. It is just part of the creative destruction of capitalism that ultimately offers consumers another choice, and if it becomes popular, that is because consumers view it as a superior value.

The difference is, Uber, Zoom, and Zappos are low-risk, repeatable operations. If you take an Uber instead of a taxicab and it's a horrible experience—the driver is a jerk who doesn't know where to go, the car is unsanitary and in poor repair, the app fails to pinpoint your location, or whatever—you're out thirty bucks, and you never use the service again. If you don't like the shoes, you never order another pair from Zappos and instead head back to your local shoe emporium. You're not doomed by one bad experience.

Experimenting with straightening teeth is something you do once in your life—you hope. A poor experience can't simply be returned for your money back or shrugged off with the consolation that you'll make a better choice next time—because there won't be a next time (unless you slink into my office forlornly to try again). The consumer experience involves not merely a pair of shoes or a videoconference; at risk is your oral health and, by extension, your overall health. It is not my turf that I am protecting; it is my patients.

I am a business owner who is always seeking new ways to grow my business and studying new products and procedures that might benefit patients and increase revenue. I admire companies that bring a great new idea to market. If I felt that mail-order orthodontics was a viable and safe alternative for my patients, I would invest in them and offer my services directly to them. We would cut out the middleman and sell direct to consumers. That's brilliant—for Amazon. They sell stuff. It's not brilliant at all for the oral health of individual patients, biological creatures endowed by their creator with infinite variability. Your oral health can't be boiled down to a shoe size, a meeting time, or a location and destination. There is so much potential for harm in these mail-order services that I could never invest in them knowing I could be contributing to hurting people, the very antithesis of my work's mission. Investing in a company in this field would keep me up at night and ultimately soil my reputation.

So if I am protecting turf, that is the turf I am protecting.

EVERY TEAM NEEDS A QUARTERBACK

When a patient is treated with Invisalign or any other clear aligner, the orthodontist is playing the role of quarterback all along the way. Sure, computer software scans the teeth, and an algorithm predicts their movement. That is necessary but not sufficient. The quarterback still must execute the play call and adjust on the fly as the play unfolds.

While a mail-order company ships the first aligner to their customer, I examine my patient and test the fit of the first aligner. It is paramount that the first one fit exactly right, or the negative consequences will ripple through the entire treatment. If you are driving to a location and you make a wrong turn out of the parking lot, continuing down the street in that direction will just get you farther from your destination. (Sorry, I have mixed metaphors a bit there.) My judgment is critical right at the beginning to ensure that everything is proceeding according to plan, a value add out of the reach of a mail-order operation.

Moreover, humans are not static entities like furniture. A yearlong plan might be perfect at the moment of design but no longer appropriate six months later. On almost every Invisalign patient I see, we make a midcourse adjustment somewhere along the line to ensure proper functioning. If we need to make some space because teeth have moved in slight variation from expectations, I might sand down a tooth. If teeth are lining up unevenly, I might add a glue glob atop a tooth so the aligner attaches to it and slowly yanks it toward the center of the bite over time. If a patient breaks a tooth and needs a crown, the aligners will no longer fit properly and the whole process must be started over with new scans and new aligners from that point onward. Occasionally, interim events such as growing bones, trauma to the mouth, or episodic commitment to the aligner prevent the teeth from making the progress predicted by the algorithm. In that case, we might need to repeat a few steps. For that we would print out some new aligners and allow the patient to make up lost ground. None of that is possible in the mail-order universe that purports to save money by cutting out the trained professional and his or her considerable judgments.

The clear aligner revolution is built on the foundation that tooth movement can be predicted by combining algorithms and artificial intelligence that has learned from the millions of past cases. The system has become remarkably good at these projections. Nonetheless, human variability is infinite, and projections are not guarantees. Some judgment is almost always going to be required.

THE ORTHODONTIST'S IMPACT ON COMPLIANCE

As I noted last chapter, compliance is an issue with Invisalign, particularly with adults. There are many reasons why individuals do or don't adhere to the protocols that optimize results. I am sure entire psychology PhD theses have been written about intrinsic versus extrinsic motivation, the value of reward versus punishment in promoting positive behavior, and all that. If you are interested in those topics, I advise you to read a book on psychology, not on orthodontics. I believe in hiring the right expert for the job, and I do not

There are no smiling faces in a faceless mail-order system, which continues sending aligners irrespective of whether the customer has been wearing the previous batch.

purport to be an expert in psychology, even after five children and thousands of patients.

That said, one psychological construct we know is at work with clear aligners—we know because we see it—is that nothing boosts compliance quite like an upcoming orthodontist visit. Put simply, people are embarrassed to fail the modest test of whether they can comply with the order to wear their appliance twenty-two hours daily. Knowing they will see not just the orthodontist but a whole staff of warm, positive, encouraging people, administrative and clinical, is a powerful motivator to follow the plan. No one wants to let down all those smiling faces. There are no smiling faces in a faceless mail-order system, which continues sending aligners irrespective of whether the customer has been wearing the previous batch.

There is one more complication to consider when researching mail-order orthodontics: sometimes what a patient really needs is more than just straightening the front teeth. Sometimes that is a very bad call that can have disastrous consequences for them. I respect the choice of patients who have lived full, healthy lives with whatever arrangements of teeth they have but would like to improve their smile. The full orthodontic treatment, enduring braces or aligners for eighteen months and spending thousands of dollars, is overkill for them. That is understandable, and as I have said, we are happy to provide this service, which is faster and less expensive than the full regimen of orthodontic care. Part of our business ethic is to provide our patients with the full array of options, make my recommendation if doing so can be helpful, and accept their choice. I won't agree to do harm to a patient, but I don't tell adults how to live or what decisions to make for their children.

That said, correctable problems, left unaddressed, can cause harm. A patient with a significant malocclusion in the back teeth can cause themselves jaw and neck pain, headaches, problems chewing food that causes stomach upset, and a flood of health issues that could have been averted with orthodontic treatment. Left untreated, the malocclusion can also undermine any smile-straightening efforts. By straightening the front teeth but not the back, the front teeth will, over time, compensate for the malocclusion, leaving the patient with nice straight buck teeth and a poor bite. The mail-order company will claim success, time will diffuse responsibility for the new problem, and the customer will never know that their issues, developed years later, resulted from their choice to cut out the expert who could have steered them to a better choice.

In the next chapter, we will explore all the effects braces have during the months that they are actually on teeth, with particular attention on staining, a common and avoidable problem.

TAKEAWAYS

→ DIY orthodontics is capitalizing on the Invisalign revolution and suggesting that a computer can diagnose an incorrect smile and create a treatment plan as well as an orthodontist can. These mail-order operations narrowly limit themselves to mild issues with front teeth only and promise merely to straighten them.

→ When you sign up for one of these mail-order systems, don't expect any guidance from them. If the aligners don't feel right, there is no way to determine whether you have them on wrong, they weren't designed correctly, or there is some other problem.

→ The ratings of these mail-order systems are so bad that if an orthodontist had half as many negative reviews, he or she would be considered incompetent and quickly lose business. There are a variety of reasons that a professional, educated, clinically trained orthodontist who meets you and sees your teeth will create a more beautiful smile nearly every time as opposed to a computer somewhere.

→ Given the narrow scope of mail-order orthodontics, they are not saving customers any money. Your local orthodontist likely will perform the same limited service for roughly the same cost and do a significantly better job in the process.

→ Many of these companies direct customers to their nearest center to develop a scan of their teeth, which will be used to build a treatment plan. If you don't live in a big city, the nearest center could be a hundred miles away or more. They also don't involve a physical exam or an x-ray of your mouth. It would be considered malpractice if an orthodontist treated you without these two. A physical exam and an x-ray can rule out a long list of health issues and problems that might undermine a straightening regimen. When issues arise after using a mail-order aligner system, customers have no recourse.

→ If anything changes in your mouth between the time the scan is done and receipt of your last aligner, there is no way to adjust the treatment. Under an orthodontist's care, that is easily solved.

➡ Cosmetic orthodontics are not like buying shoes or hailing a ride. A customer only gets one chance to get it right and is gambling thousands of dollars on people they never meet.

➡ There are many situations in which patients only want to correct their smile, but they really need something else. Their health may be at risk.

CHAPTER 8

"DO BRACES REALLY STAIN TEETH?"

WHEN YOU WALK into our orthodontic office in Northern Utah to begin your journey with braces, one of the warm, encouraging professionals you will meet is Jennifer (not her real name), one of our clinical assistants. Living with braces is a new way of life, a little different than living without them, because, to state the obvious, you don't ordinarily walk around twenty-four hours a day with metal tugging on your teeth. Even in the case of clear aligners, you're still wearing a plastic mouthpiece almost all your waking hours. In either case, the appliance is slowly persuading your teeth to shift into a new alignment, which means there is constant tension on your mouth and jaws. Additionally, brushing and flossing correctly will simultaneously become more difficult and significantly more critical. That is where Jennifer comes in.

Jennifer is our primary patient educator. She explains to patients how to brush and floss, what to eat and drink and what not to, why teeth stain and how to avoid it, and the general care and maintenance of braces. Jennifer uses graphs and charts and pedagogical aids like a set of tooth models—and cute little aphorisms that make it all easy to remember—to the point where she is the company expert on patient compliance. Frankly, she should be writing this section of the book, because she has the patter memorized and has already encountered every off-the-wall question one could conjure—and put it to rest with a pithy response. As it is my book, I'll simply pass along Jennifer's wise counsel.

Jennifer's expertise does not come entirely from the office: she knows firsthand of what she speaks. As we will discuss in a subsequent chapter, one of the highlights of Jennifer's life was the day her husband surprised her with a Christmas gift of the orthodontic care she had always wished she had experienced as a child. She was in her thirties at the time. I'll never forget how she beamed the day her braces … went on! It was the satisfied smile most patients flash when their braces come off, but Jennifer was so excited about finally getting her teeth straightened that she was elated just to begin the process. Evidently the experience was extremely positive for her, because after her treatment she came to work with us and has been a huge asset to the practice for years. So she has lived through brushing with an electric toothbrush and other oddly shaped tools, cutting apples before eating them, chewing candy with the inside of her mouth, and all the other fun stuff required to maintain the integrity of metal braces and ensure good dental hygiene.

Thanks to Jennifer's masterful tutorials, we have a high compliance rate. Patients leave on that first day with a very clear idea of how they should be treating their braces and their teeth, and if they forget, she has included cheat sheets in the kit they take home with them. All this is a very long preamble to the acknowledgment that the following instructions on how to care for your mouth with braces grew out of a collaboration between me and my staff, most notably Jennifer.

THE SCIENCE BEHIND CLEANING TEETH

In your mouth, at this very moment, live billions of bacteria. Don't feel bad: billions of bacteria live in my mouth, too, and everyone else's, for that matter. Most of these bacteria are either harmless or beneficial, helping to break down food, create saliva, and perform a host of other oral functions. Among these bacteria are twenty-five

Brush and floss. There is no substitute.

different kinds of streptococci, one of which, *Streptococcus mutans*, is the main culprit in tooth decay. The favorite meal of *Strep mutans* is sugar, which it digests to form a sticky substance that adheres to teeth and produces acid that breaks down tooth enamel. When a significant amount of dental decay occurs, it can lead to cavities and other issues that we are all trying to avoid. Limiting your sugar intake can help mitigate the effects of *Strep mutans*, but the only foolproof method of fighting tooth decay is to brush and floss your teeth regularly.

Brush and floss. There is no substitute.

Even if you do avoid sugar and follow directions to brush and floss, you know when you visit the dentist that you may nonetheless have plaque, which is *Strep mutans* and its accompanying detritus, like an unwelcome visitor squatting in your house with all their baggage. You may have experienced a fuzzy feeling on your teeth, as if they are wearing a sweater. That is a serious buildup of plaque. Recall how clean and sparkly your teeth feel after a dental cleaning with the gritty cleaning agent that scrapes plaque off the teeth. Keep in mind that it feels great immediately after the treatment, but it is all downhill from there. From the moment the hygienist and dentist are done with the cleaning, the process begins again, and the bacteria starts munching on sugar, replicating and producing acid to harm your teeth.

Brushing teeth fights the plaque by tearing the *Strep mutans* from the surface of teeth. But toothbrush bristles have a hard time entering every dental nook and cranny, particularly in the wide, creviced surface of molars, which are most susceptible to cavities. Even when the brush is scientifically engineered to contact hard-to-reach parts of the teeth, we don't always use perfect form when brushing and can miss those areas. Spaces between teeth are nearly impossible to reach with a toothbrush even when brushed correctly, which is why dentists and orthodontists recommend everyone floss as a regular element of their morning and evening ablutions. Flossing and brushing also keep plaque out of gums, which hold the teeth in place and can become infected and inflamed by the same processes. So brushing and flossing keep periodontists happy too.

Children's teeth also benefit from the fluoride treatment of public drinking water. The fluoride bonds with growing enamel, making it harder and more resistant to decay. Studies have found a 35 percent decline in tooth decay among children drinking fluoridated water. There is no empirical evidence of benefit for adults, whose tooth enamel has already hardened.[12]

Some years ago I was the presenter in a continuing education course for dental hygienists. Like many licensed healthcare professionals, hygienists must attend periodic courses to keep their skills current and learn new techniques, practices, and science. In the course of the discussion, I asked the group what I could do as an orthodontist to enhance the oral hygiene of the public and make their job easier. I was surprised by the level of consensus in their answer, which was to recommend to all my patients that they use electric toothbrushes.

---

12   Zipporah Iheozor-Ejiofor et al., "Water Fluoridation for the Prevention of Dental Caries," *Cochrane Database of Systematic Reviews* 6 (June 18, 2015): https://doi.org//10.1002/14651858.CD010856.pub2.

Since then, we have included a high-quality electric toothbrush in the materials we provide for every patient who comes in for braces. Electric toothbrushes are easier to use than manual brushes, particularly for patients with limited mobility in their hands. They add vibrating action that is not dependent on hand movement and have thus proven more adept at removing plaque. Many electric toothbrushes come with built-in timers, which keep people brushing longer and increasing the number of surfaces covered. You don't have to be old or infirm to benefit from an electric toothbrush.

Of course, nearly all my patients have one thing in common that is not shared by the public at large—they are wearing braces or aligners, which is to say they have special challenges in brushing and flossing at the same time that maintaining good oral health is particularly critical. For the millions of North Americans who are or will be wearing braces, here are Jennifer's brushing, flossing, eating, and tooth care instructions.

BRUSHING AND FLOSSING WITH BRACES

Picture in your mind a set of teeth with metal brackets glued tightly to the front and a wire running through all the brackets. It is pretty clear how attempting to brush teeth in that configuration would be a daunting and time-consuming task. The challenge, however, must be met, because people with braces who don't brush and floss meticulously risk staining their teeth permanently, which somewhat undermines the whole idea of straightening teeth and beautifying a smile. Even for those wearing aligners, who are not challenged by a metal appliance blocking the way, brushing and flossing, not to mention rinsing the mouth and the aligner, are critical to maintaining the oral health conditions for orthodontic success.

If you were in the chair at our practice, Jennifer would, after greeting you and melting your heart with her personal warmth and empathy, hold up a set of models and instruct you that, for the next year or two, you would be brushing your teeth differently. First, she would point out the particular importance of angling the brush so that you are making contact with your gums. The gum line is most susceptible to infection and must be cleaned methodically every time the teeth are brushed. With braces, the head of the toothbrush doesn't have much room to maneuver, and the brush won't hit the gum line unless the bristles are intentionally angled toward the gums—that is, downward on the bottom teeth and upward on the top teeth. Patients following just that one piece of advice are already much of the way to good oral hygiene with braces.

As I mentioned, this is most often going to be accomplished with the electric toothbrush we provide for patients, at least when they are brushing at home. Irrespective of the type of brush, manual or electric, the key remains complete dental coverage and angling the bristles toward the gums. For after-meal brushing, the same strategies can be applied with a manual toothbrush. Brushing after every meal is a great practice but not one that we push. We are realistic about how willing people are to enter a public bathroom, such as a workplace or restaurant bathroom, and begin brushing their teeth as traffic flows in and out.

When this discussion is happening with children—and that is our primary audience here—Jennifer will ask the parent to model the behavior she has just recommended. We're generally talking to a mom, so when Mom acts out what Jennifer has described and demonstrates to the child the proper technique, she is both demonstrating to her child the technique involved and also lending her imprimatur to its consistent application. We have found that this small act both aids understanding and promotes compliance, especially after we tell Mom that failing to follow our directions could result in stains on her child's teeth after she has spent thousands of dollars to straighten them.

It is pretty evident that a normal toothbrush is not going to get under the brace wire or near the brackets. For that, Jennifer demonstrates use of the proxy brush, or what she calls the Christmas tree brush. It is much smaller than a normal toothbrush and sticks out straight from the handle in an upside-down V shape that resembles a Christmas tree. This brush can be slid under the wire and used to brush around the brackets and under the wire. This is the area most likely to stain from poor brushing, so Jennifer emphasizes the importance of strict adherence to that added regimen.

Given the complexity of brushing with braces that is new to all new patients, we highly recommend measuring the results. There are two ways to do this: (1) wait until teeth stain and cavities emerge to determine that the results were poor, or (2) chew on pink disclosing tablets that light up the areas that haven't been brushed. I can't speak for all orthodontists, but in our office, we opt for the method that doesn't cause pain, suffering, disfigurement, and further dental work. Consequently, Jennifer demonstrates to patients how the pink tablets work. Following their new dental regimen, the patient swishes around the pink tablets in their mouth and spits it out. Then they smile in front of a mirror and are inevitably horrified about how much of their mouth is pink, pinker, and near red. The darker, the worse, giving patients a clear indication of

Brushing without flossing is like soaping your car without rinsing it, or cooking the turkey without carving it, or … well, the point is, it is a job half-done.

how much more diligent they need to be about brushing. We often will do the first course right here in the office, which always leads to a second brushing and so on until they get positive feedback. We find that piloting the pink tablets in the office may itself be sufficient, because it plants in the child's mind how much more industrious their brushing has to be. We do give them a small supply, and I hope they use it and improve their technique over time, but even if they don't, that practice session often sticks with them. It is not quite like touching a hot stove once, but the theory is the same.

Brushing without flossing is like soaping your car without rinsing it, or cooking the turkey without carving it, or … well, the point is, it is a job half-done. Necessary but not sufficient. No matter how well anyone brushes, there is no way to get the bristles in between the teeth, and that goes double for anyone wearing braces. Flossing remains critical to good oral health, except that with braces, as you can imagine, it is doubly difficult. Jennifer knows that firsthand, which is why she introduces patients to the angled flossing stick. It comes in a variety of shapes and configurations under brand names like Plackers and DenTek and others. The one we provide can slide under the wire in the correct position to glide between the teeth and remove food and plaque from those areas. For the occasional slot that even the angled stick cannot access, the type we provide comes with a flossing pic inside the handle—it's basically a plastic toothpick—that can be bent into position to reach those recalcitrant areas, usually in the very back. Jennifer admonishes our patients—in a way that makes it sound like both a compliment and an honor—to floss every time they brush, which had better be at least twice daily.

Next, Jennifer introduces the patient to the world of rubbing, chafing, and scraping that all brace-wearing people inhabit. As a former resident, Jennifer is equipped to lay out the welcome mat and host them on their journey. With metal on and around teeth, there will likely be occasions when some part of the appliance is rubbing, poking, or scraping against some part of the patient's mouth. They are the facts of braces life, and experiencing them simply ushers the user into a global club of millions. The good news is that there are some simple solutions. That is where the wax box comes in.

If you have never worn braces, you are unlikely to have ever made the acquaintance of the wax box, but it is a great friend to those so encumbered. Inside the wax box are little strips of wax that can be easily rolled into balls. The wax holds its form in the box, but the warmth of our fingers melts it a bit and makes it extremely pliable. As long as the bracket or wire is dry, the wax can be applied to the offending metal to form a soft cushion between the brace and the gum, lip, tongue, or whatever. For patients with an overbite, it may be necessary to apply the entire strip of wax across the brackets. The wax comes in a variety of palate-pleasing flavors like mint and cinnamon, but no one should mistake that for an invitation to swallow. Like toothpaste, wax is not food, and ingesting it should be avoided. Still, like toothpaste, swallowing is likely inevitable and unremarkable as long as it is kept to a minimum. I imagine if someone ate an entire wax box, they might get a stomachache, but I have no empirical evidence of that.

Our experience with all this is the following: adults, who tend to be highly motivated to have a positive experience, have no trouble following our directions. Children who make any effort at all do a pretty good job as well. These two groups never get stains on their teeth; in fact, their dental health generally improves as they become more focused on the need to brush and floss every single tooth every single morning and every single night. Then there are the children who don't care and whose parents either don't make much effort to convince them otherwise or who try mightily but don't succeed. These kids usually have other mental, emotional, or behavioral issues that transcend the orthodontist's office, and pretty soon they have stains on their teeth. I can use a whitening or bleaching agent on the offending teeth that mitigates the stain, but it is not a substitute for avoiding the problem. Once teeth stain from poor dental hygiene, the only way to completely remove it is a trip to the dentist for a filling.

EATING AND DRINKING WITH BRACES

Care for teeth with braces is about more than brushing and flossing. After all, as we were just discussing with respect to stains, prevention is better than attempting to cure. Jennifer's tutorial does not end there; it is just getting revved up. Next, she instructs our patients what and how to eat.

Let me just intervene here with a side note: if you are going to wear braces, there are foods that, in a perfect world, you would simply avoid. The fact is, no one in the world should ever consume soda. Cola particularly is an industrial solvent with a pH of 2.4—that is, it is just slightly less acidic than hydrochloric acid, a highly corrosive liquid that damages skin on contact. Regular cola is so loaded with refined sugar that one sixteen-ounce can alone exceeds the recommended daily sugar limit for women. Sugary soft drinks are responsible in part for our nation's epidemic of diabetes, obesity, and general poor health. You probably know that and probably drink soda. I do now and then, even though I'm a medical professional and my specialty is teeth, which are especially harmed by sugar. So if I could wave a magic wand, my patients would never drink soda whether they have braces or not.

If I may continue my wand waving for just a moment, I would also prohibit my patients who are getting braces from eating gooey candy like Tootsie Rolls and Gummy Bears. They gum up the works and take hours, literally hours, to extract from every bracket. I would demand that they lay off the hard candy like Jawbreakers and the crunchy stuff like chips, pretzels, and granola bars. Things like that have a nasty habit of breaking the braces and requiring repair at the most inopportune times, like Christmas Eve, the day of my son's wedding, or the day of the patient's wedding. My patients would only eat meat, fruits, vegetables, and beans if I were king of the world and my orthodontic wish were my patients' command.

Alas, that is not reality. Not only are people going to eat and drink what they want, but they're not going to keep track of what is on the good list and what isn't. Or at least many people won't. I have had some patients who have told me that they would simply eliminate whatever foods I recommended they eliminate. But they are so few and far between that they could socially distance inside a Bloodmobile. Knowing that my patients would respond to such commands with the same bemusement my kids do, we dispatch Jennifer to help our patients eat what they want safely.

Jennifer, bless her, doesn't care about all that. She sat in that same chair today's patients sit in and knows what they are thinking: give up Starbursts, popcorn, diet Sprite? No way. I want straight teeth, not admittance into a monastery. She understands and advises them to eat whatever they like. Yes, eat it all—crunchy, chewy, hard, and gooey, it's all okay. But how you eat it—that is a different story. It's all there on the card Jennifer hands every patient.

We want our patients to be able to eat foods like a crisp apple. Even with braces, patients can eat apples but must cut them up first. Taking a big bite out of an apple is a nearly foolproof prescription for broken braces. That is Jennifer starting slow. Then she moves on to ice. Patients can still have ice in their drinks and can even consume the ice—but they can't chew it. Ice accommodates people with braces by melting, so we suggest they just suck on the ice.

Next comes the sticky stuff. This is the part of the discussion I can't bear to hear. Jennifer calls this the "ooey-gooeys," things like caramel, saltwater taffy, fruit roll-ups, and jujubes. She tells patients to suck on them, too, and avoid chewing for the reasons I noted previously. There is no amount of brushing, flossing, and picking that can reliably remove these sticky, sugar-filled concoctions. You simply don't want your teeth involved in the act of consuming these things.

For the hard stuff like lollipops, cough drops, peanuts, and popcorn, people with braces need to be very careful. You know how peanuts and popcorn lodge in your teeth long after eating them; the problem becomes more acute with a metal appliance on your teeth. Jennifer instructs our patients to suck on them as much as possible, then chew them with the inside of their teeth, maintaining vigilance against getting them on the outside of the teeth where the braces sit. If a piece of food does get into the bracket, we recommend immediately dislodging it with a proxy brush or flosser. "Don't use your finger," Jennifer advises, "because a finger can break a bracket. We're trying not to break our brackets."

We do advise against eating one group of foods altogether for the first few days or weeks until patients get a good feel for how to eat them. Foods falling into the crunchy category—chips, pretzels, granola bars, and so on—should be avoided until the patient acclimates to their braces. Ultimately, these also need to be sucked on to soften them before chewing with the inside of the teeth.

The sugary drinks that I alluded to previously, which include sodas of all kinds and fruit juices, obviously do not require any special arrangements to consume with braces. Guzzling them is no harder with braces than without, but it is important that patients at the very least rinse out their mouths after consuming anything sugary to wash the substance off the surface of teeth and out of the oral cavity. This does not apply to "diet" drinks that use sugar substitutes, which generally do not promote bacteria growth to the same extent as the glucose found in most desserts. They are, however, very acidic and should be avoided just like their sugary cousins.

Finally, Jennifer does have to lay the hammer down on one food in particular because there is just no way to use this item as directed and enjoy a happy experience with braces. Anyone beginning a treatment with metal braces must steel themselves for a future without bubble gum. Chewing sugarless gum can be a great way to relieve aching in the teeth and stimulate the production of saliva that keeps the mouth clean and removes sugar. I heartily endorse my patients chew sugarless gum if they so choose. But bubble gum, whose sole purpose is to exit the mouth and create a balloon of stretched confection that collapses across the teeth, is absolutely verboten. Patients risk a face full of resin and a return trip to the orthodontist if they chew bubble gum and blow bubbles. Any such patient will discover, when they return to our office with an orthodontic appliance coated in gum, that they will have to have their braces replaced. Far worse, they will know the shame of disappointing Jennifer. Believe me, there is no worse feeling than letting down this angel of mercy who has specifically forbidden the very behavior you have practiced.

That is the eating-and-drinking tutorial, which we reemphasize the first few times children return to our office. We prefer to find out sooner rather than later that there is going to be a compliance issue with it so we can institute some preventive measures, most notably having a word with Mom. Most patients make a sincere effort to eat and drink carefully and care for their teeth; after all, they are spending time and money to improve the way their teeth function and look. We have had a handful of notable exceptions, one of which jumps to mind as the textbook failure in that regard. Unfortunately, this involved a family that did not share the motivation I just mentioned.

SOME PEOPLE JUST CAN'T MANAGE IT

We sometimes take on patients who present to us with dental hygiene issues from the start, knowing that this is a risky proposition. Many Americans are not knowledgeable about proper dental care and see a dentist only when there is an issue, like a cavity that is causing pain. The problem is often not that they are uninterested or unwilling to care for their teeth but that either they aren't aware that dental care must be practiced prophylactically and consistently or there are barriers to doing so, most notably a lack of dental insurance or other resources to pay for care. Often, families like these can become good stewards of their own oral hygiene once we educate them about the importance of brushing, flossing, and visiting a dentist regularly for checkups and point them to the resources available to help them.

We encountered one such patient, a fourteen-year-old boy with a host of dental issues. His teeth were covered in plaque, and his gums looked like they had never been brushed. They were red and puffy, to the point that I could make them bleed simply by blowing air onto them. This was a young man in dire need of orthodontic care, but he first required some serious attention from a dentist. I recommended to his mom that he see a dentist before we embarked on orthodontic care.

At our office, we accept patients who will pay for their services with Medicaid because we believe everyone deserves access to orthodontic care. It turned out that he had sixteen cavities that required attention, which they received, and after a few months, he was back in our chair. It was important at that point that we had an honest discussion with him and his mother about the importance of maintaining good oral health if his orthodontic treatment was going to succeed, and they appeared committed.

We went forward with treatment, and all was well for months, but eventually his compliance began to slip, and the condition of his teeth deteriorated. His mother was understandably frustrated but was unable to convince him to attend to his oral hygiene needs every morning and night. It got so bad that about two-thirds of the way through his treatment, we were forced to remove the braces.

If I put myself in his shoes, it is easy to see why his motivation slipped. At the two-thirds point in almost anyone's orthodontic treatment, the functional issues with their teeth have been relieved and most of the straightening is done. While the professionals in my office could see what was missing when we removed his braces, from his vantage point his teeth were straight and his biting and chewing were improved. In the short-run thinking of a (now) fifteen-year-old boy, he had gotten his money's worth and wasn't much concerned with the marginal difference we wanted to continue making with his smile. The path for rationalizing his lack of effort was well paved.

Additionally, it was easy to get his money's worth because his family was not paying for this service—Medicaid was. What we regard as an expensive failure, he viewed through a different lens. It was free, and the results were great. Of course, he is going to have ongoing issues with his teeth, and if he continues down the road he is on, they are going to rot, fall out, and give him significant problems by the time he is thirty-five. But he is not the first fifteen-year-old to whom his fate twenty years hence does not mean very much.

It is worth reiterating that we have had the great fortune to meet dozens of children from families of modest financial means who relied on Medicaid to transform the functioning of their teeth and provide an artistic smile. Most of them, even those who present to us with suboptimal dental hygiene habits when they arrive, learn the correct regimen and adapt quickly. We have many very happy success stories that fit that general outline, but it is the one failure that sticks in our craw and led to long discussions among our staff about how to better manage.

WHAT HAPPENS WHEN BRACES BREAK

After all that, after Jennifer's magnificent performance, with visual aids and folksy maxims delivered with the noncaloric sweetness of stevia, patients nonetheless manage to chomp down on something that breaks, disassembles, cracks, twists, unhinges, or otherwise makes the braces inoperable; we have a regimen for that. If a bracket breaks off a tooth in the back and slides back and forth on the wire, she tells patients it can usually wait until the next appointment. The brackets are doing less work the farther back they go. Brackets that break on the front teeth usually must be repaired right away, which means an unscheduled trip to see us. Repair in these cases precludes some of the backtracking that occurs when the braces cease their work of nudging teeth into the desired positions. When brackets dislodge from teeth, we do ask patients to collect them and bring them to us; they are generally not broken, simply detached. Many a time, patients have fished their bracket out of a sandwich or soup bowl and deposited it into a baggie for easy transport back to the mother ship.

The wire, which is the most delicate and exposed element of the appliance, is also the most crucial. A broken wire must be repaired for a number of reasons. The wire is responsible for all the tension that moves teeth, so a broken wire means the entire system is inoperable. Broken wires are also an injury hazard because the broken end is sharp and can puncture a cheek, lip, gum, or tongue. There is no best case among those four, so we advise patients with broken wires to come in immediately.

CARE FOR CLEAR ALIGNERS

The care for clear aligners is vastly different and significantly easier. We do not unleash Jennifer upon aligner patients because the instructions are so easy to sketch out that even an orthodontist can do it. We tell our patients whose orthodontic care involves aligners that ideally they would brush their teeth and the aligner after every meal. One of the beauties of aligners is that they are easily removed for, among other things, tooth brushing and flossing. Wearing a device over teeth for twenty-two hours daily does increase the importance of good dental hygiene, but we're also realistic about whether people are going to brush their teeth or their aligner at work in the middle of the day. We tell patients that if they can't bring themselves to brush after lunch, at least brush teeth and aligners in the morning and at night, which is already most people's habit, and vigorously rinse out the aligner after meals so that food and residue do not accumulate on them and on the teeth inside them.

The other problem with aligners, associated with the great advantage that they can be removed, is losing them. The trick we teach our patients is to consider only two homes for the aligner—in your mouth or in its case. Because aligners are clear, they are masters at hide-and-seek. If they are placed down on a surface, they have a habit of disappearing. They also like to conceal themselves in napkins where mildly embarrassed users wrap them during meals outside the house—whether at school or during the workday. Forgotten in the napkin, they naturally get scooped up and added to the dirty dishes for removal into the trash. No one wants to sift through garbage to find an aligner and then return it to their mouth. That is why we tell patients that if the aligner is not in your mouth (or being washed), it should be in its little round hockey puck–sized case, which fits in a pocket or purse and is less likely to avoid detection or find its way to the refuse.

I think you would be surprised by the low rate of loss of aligners. We have never had a patient lose a replacement aligner (i.e., no one has ever lost two in the space of a couple of months). One young patient did lose his entire set of eight aligners—well, seven, because one was in his mouth—immediately upon leaving our office. We gave him a little time, and he eventually found them long before he was ready for the next in the series. When patients lose their aligner, we will generally order a new one quickly. If they are nearly done with it, we will instruct them to ascend to the next in the series. If the aligner is lost because it hasn't been worn in days or even weeks, then we have a whole other problem and likely need to go backward and retrace our steps. And have a little heart-to-heart with our patient.

WHAT IS AN ORTHODONTIC EMERGENCY?

In three decades of treating patients, I have experienced one true emergency—when a patient swallowed the wire of their metal brace. The irony of this is that once the situation enters the realm of true emergency, I am not the kind of doctor you want caring for you. That particular patient went to the emergency room, where the physician x-rayed his gastrointestinal tract and decided to leave it alone and track its progress. The patient either digested or excreted it, because it was never an issue, much to my relief as well as his. Patients have lost brackets in ways that suggested they probably swallowed them—the rubber bands, too—but they are small enough that it is unlikely to present any danger, other than perhaps a mild stomachache.

The kinds of orthodontic emergencies that we talk about are not true emergencies, but we certainly feel obliged to react immediately. That primarily involves a broken wire sticking into a body part and causing pain and distress. If you call the office after hours you will be directed to call an emergency number, which is my personal cell phone. In most cases, using Jennifer's wax trick takes care of the problem until the next workday, but occasionally immediate action is necessary, and I will offer to meet the patient at our office. Clipping a wire literally takes ten seconds. If a back bracket falls off, exposing the wire to the mouth, reattaching the bracket takes three minutes. On those rare occasions that a change in the brace is caused by trauma, there is the added time factor of an x-ray and more careful attention to the health of the patient's mouth. Our mouths bleed profusely; it is important for me to carefully determine whether serious damage has occurred. The worst cases I have seen involved teeth being dislodged—often preserved by the braces—in which case the teeth must be put back in place manually under anesthesia.

THE LEGEND OF KISSING WITH BRACES

You've seen or heard the legend of teenagers locked in a loving embrace—literally locked because their braces have intertwined and they are bound to each other by mouth in mortification until someone, usually stifling guffaws, patiently disconnects them. It's a pretty funny cautionary tale that has served recalcitrant dating partners for a century.

It's just not true.

I mean, theoretically braces could become locked, just as theoretically alligators could be living in the sewers underneath New York, having been flushed down toilets as babies by hundreds of disgusted parents. Each story has just enough plausibility to be believable without actually being true. In three decades of professional service, I have never heard of a single case and do not know another orthodontist or dentist with firsthand knowledge of a single case. Nonetheless, I do my best to perpetuate the myth to keep rowdy teenagers from behaving badly. I'm the father of four boys, so I know the value of maintaining decorum with a little hyperbole.

There—you now have the manual for care of teeth and braces during orthodontic treatment. Next, we'll review what a bargain orthodontic care is and reveal something surprising: as an orthodontist, I know almost nothing about which patients are paying and which are in arrears, how much they pay, or what payment plan they have chosen.

TAKEAWAYS

➡ Taking care of your teeth and gums by brushing and flossing is important under ordinary circumstances; it's even more important with braces.

➡ Braces make it difficult to brush and floss assiduously, so patients are provided with an electric toothbrush, a proxy brush, and an angled flossing stick that comes with a toothpick.

➡ There are certain foods that people with braces really shouldn't eat—sticky, gooey, and hard snacks. We know they are going to eat them anyway, so we provide detailed instructions on how to eat these foods so they don't break their braces.

➡ Crunchy snacks, like chips and pretzels, should be avoided the first few days until the patient gets acclimated to eating with braces.

➡ Chewing sugarless gum is good for people with braces because it cleans the mouth and relieves the ache. Bubble gum is prohibited because bubbles pop and can ruin the braces.

➡ When braces break, it is usually not an emergency. If back brackets come off, we wait generally until the next appointment to fix them. Front brackets usually must be repaired right away, as must broken wires.

➡ Aligners don't require the same level of care but should be rinsed thoroughly after eating. When not in use, they should be stored in their case so they aren't lost.

→ The biggest emergencies related to orthodontics involve trauma to the teeth and broken wires poking the mouth. Both are relatively easily addressed. Calling my office emergency number after hours and on weekends gets patients directly to me.

→ There is no evidence that teenagers are susceptible to locking their braces when they kiss. It is theoretically possible, but I've never seen it in more than thirty years of practice.

CHAPTER 9

"BRACES ARE JUST TOO EXPENSIVE"

BACK IN THE EARLY 1980s, I got a job working for a drilling company outside Grand Junction, Colorado. I wasn't actually involved in the drilling; in fact, you could say I was the team's water boy. Drilling machines get hot and need to be cooled down with tons of water—literally tons of it. I drove the water truck, filling it up with water and bringing it to the site. Every day, back and forth from the man-made lake to the drilling site I drove. It was hot, dusty, and a little lonely, but I made good money for a college kid plus a hundred dollars per day for living expenses out in the middle of nowhere.

Some guys viewed that one hundred dollars as their ticket to luxurious living and hard partying off the job, but I was frugal and goal oriented. I slept in a tent at a KOA campground, ate food from the grocery store, and generally regarded the per diem as a savings bonus. The result was that I was socking away a lot of money, and by the end of the summer I had earned the next year's tuition plus enough extra to buy a brand-new Honda Accord. It cost me $8,000 and was by far the largest outlay of cash I had ever made up to that point in my life. Today, with inflation, a new Accord would set you back roughly $25,000, or three times as much.

The reason I mention this is that it is a good basis for comparison with braces. A set of braces purchased in the early 1980s cost about $2,500–$3,000. Today those "same" braces run roughly $4,500 in my office, less than twice as much. Relative to that Honda, the cost of orthodontic care has declined by more than a third.

I put "same" in quotation marks because the orthodontic care of the early 1980s isn't available today. The state of the art has advanced radically since then, as I have outlined in previous chapters. The materials, methods, and diagnostic tools have advanced; scanning has replaced molds; the use of preadjusted braces and direct bonding have become common; self-ligating braces have improved; lingual and ceramic braces have become options; and—the big one—we have all benefited from the clear aligner revolution. The cost for orthodontic care at my office is the same whether a patient opts for metal braces or clear aligners, which is the rough automobile equivalent of comparing the price of a Honda Accord in the early 1980s with a hybrid electric-gasoline Toyota Prius today (roughly $32,000) that pollutes less, runs silently, and gets fifty-plus miles per gallon. Orthodontic patients today are getting so much more for their money at a lower real price, and the process is more comfortable, requires fewer trips to the ortho-dontist, and produces more consistent results.

Automobiles are just one comparison point, but there are so many others. If you wanted to see your favorite musical act in 1985, you paid $15 for a ticket on average and nearly $100 today—a nearly sevenfold hike. A single-family home in an average American market that cost $82,500 in 1985 would go for $330,800 today, or four times the price. Private four-year college tuition of $5,560 in 1985 sets a family back $38,000 today, or about seven times as much. Perhaps a more apt comparison is medical care, since orthodontic treatment is more closely associated to the healthcare industry than any other. In 1985, Americans spent an average of $1,800 for medical care. That number has ballooned to more than $11,000 today, a sixfold increase. Clearly, orthodontic treatment is a relative bargain even if a family must pay the full cost, which it often does not.

In the early 1980s, when medical care was relatively affordable, insurance was something of an afterthought. No one needed to break open the 401(k) piggy bank to pay for a simple procedure, which is a good thing, because 401(k)s were just a few years old and not widespread in the early 1980s. Few people had dental insurance, and I am not aware of any insurance that would cover orthodontic treatment. Today a wide variety of dental policies cover at least some orthodontics. That $4,500 bill could be shaved to $4,000 or $2,000 or nothing. Commonly, when insurance does cover orthodontics, it covers a percentage of the cost—often 50 percent—with a maximum amount, say $1,500. In that case, the family saves $1,500 and pays $2,500 out of pocket. It is both a substantial savings and a significant commitment to the child's future.

People with beautiful smiles feel better, look better, have more confidence, and are generally happier, and we are more likely to want to be around them.

Irrespective of whether a family has dental insurance that covers orthodontic treatment or the out-of-pocket cost is three grand or five grand or more, that is a lot of money. For roughly $5,000, a family of four could take a trip to Yellowstone National Park for a week. I would much prefer to visit Yellowstone than get braces, so I understand the sacrifice families make to provide a beautiful smile for their child.

Yet millions of Americans put their children in braces for reasons I have covered previously and won't belabor here. It seems obvious, I think, to many families that the investment today in orthodontic treatment will pay off in many multiples over the course of a child's life in measurable earning power due in part to the confidence of knowing one has a brilliant smile and an attractive face. The abstract emotional benefit, which is not quantifiable, feels logarithmically larger. People with beautiful smiles feel better, look better, have more confidence, and are generally happier, and we are more likely to want to be around them. Let's return to my colleague, Jennifer, the poster adult for the emotional benefits of braces.

THE INCALCULABLE EMOTIONAL VALUE OF A SMILE

Recall that Jennifer was not a member of my staff when her husband surprised her with the Christmas present of a beautiful smile. All you husbands can imagine how fraught with danger it is to give your wife a gift that suggests she is not a perfect beauty. But Jennifer's husband knew that she felt a deep, lingering vulnerability about her teeth and had always wished her parents had fixed her smile as a child. When Jennifer opened her present, she broke down in tears of gratitude.

Jennifer describes her preorthodontic smile as "monster teeth." She had had some terrifying experiences with dentists and was wracked with a combination of anticipation and terror at the prospect of having teeth pulled and braces applied. Generally speaking, her mouth was a source of emotional pain and even shame, and while the prospect of fixing it excited her no end, it also brought sudden attention to the body part she least wanted anyone to regard. When she first appeared in our office, we laid out a plan to begin braces in a couple of weeks.

Jennifer politely rejected the plan. She was so anxious that she wanted to start right away. Two days later she had braces on her teeth.

Many people like the clear aligners or ceramic braces because they are largely invisible to those with whom they come in contact. Jennifer, on the other hand, wanted the whole world to see that she was addressing what she felt was a glaring hinderance to her beauty. Before the braces she felt that everyone who met her was blinded not by pearly white teeth but by a crooked smile. She wanted metal braces that advertised her new path, and she wanted to talk about it with everyone she knew because she was proud of what she was doing. "I just glowed. I bragged about them. I didn't care at all about the little bit of discomfort," she says. "It was life changing."

Remember, this is how she talked during the process of putting on the braces. We often hear this sort of talk when they come off, but Jennifer was over the moon just thinking about the outcome. This is like the joy a child feels knowing that her parents are taking her to Disneyland. She brags to her friends and cannot wait to go. The travel is long and arduous, but she is unfazed. This was the situation with Jennifer, a married thirtysomething adult with a child of her own.

When the braces finally came off, Jennifer did something she had tried not to do her entire life before that: she smiled. A big, bright, perfect, face-crunching, teeth-baring, lottery-winning, Colgate-commercial smile. Then she did something else new. "I wasn't a picture-taking girl," she says. "Now there are pictures of me smiling."

The experience was so powerful for her that she whisked her daughter to our office. After a childhood of thumb sucking, the child had a serious overbite that prompted classmates to call her "squirrel girl." We put braces on her, and when they came off, she cried. "I always thought I was ugly, but I'm cute!" she said. Today she is a beautiful young adult who makes her mother proud.

You can see why we could not wait to invite Jennifer to join our staff. She offers to dubious patients fervent, first-person testimony of the benefits of orthodontics and infects those patients with her enthusiasm. She is a walking billboard for our services, not because we pay her or because it helps the business but because braces transformed her life, and she wants to share her joy with everyone else whose smile could use some help. The point here is that, for Jennifer, our treatment was priceless, something that improves her life every day. Her only regret is that she hadn't done it three decades earlier.

AN INVESTMENT IN YOUR CHILD'S FUTURE

As I mentioned in chapter 3, the research demonstrating a correlation between physical attractiveness and a host of positive financial and emotional outcomes is so robust as to be undeniable. Straightening teeth is an investment in a child's future that research proves will pay off even before accounting for how much better a child will feel about him- or herself. Remember the research by Dove soap—that nearly three-quarters of girls aged fifteen to seventeen have skipped school or avoided other normal daily activities that involve interactions with people because they feel bad about their looks. It's a vivid picture of the emotional price paid for low self-esteem regarding physical attractiveness.

I have fully subscribed to this belief with my own family. All five of my children, in varying stages of need, spent time in the chair in my office for their own experience with braces. Like any father, I wanted to give my kids the best chance to succeed in life that I could.

The value of great orthodontic care goes well beyond the cosmetic and its emotional ramifications, as we discussed in chapter 3. Teeth must be aligned correctly to facilitate biting and chewing, the first two functions in the digestion chain that allow us to extract nutrients from food and power our bodies' engines. Recall the studies demonstrating how the inability to chew adequately causes a host of digestion issues that lead to a cascade of difficulties involving almost every bodily function. Misalignment can also cause musculoskeletal pain and dysfunction, like disease of the TM joint that connects the jaw; speech difficulties; ear, nose, and throat problems; and much more. You might remember our patient Teddy, whose orthodontic dysfunction limited his diet to easily swallowed foods and prevented him from diversifying his diet to include foods that require biting, like corn on the cob and apples. Because all our bodily systems are integrated and interdependent, trouble with teeth and jaws can and do negatively affect every aspect of physical life. How much is it worth to avoid even one hazard on that list?

Among the many benefits of recent advances in teeth-straightening technology is the plethora of options available to families at various price points. For those focused solely on cost, we can straighten front teeth for a fraction of the usual cost of braces. Clear aligners often cost more than metal braces, though in my office we charge the same amount for both. Ceramic braces, lingual braces, and a host of other options allow patients and their families to customize the cost-benefit relationship that works best for them.

You might be surprised to know that, although I am generally aware of the price of my services, I am very disconnected from the financial end of the operation, and this is not uncommon for orthodontists across the nation. We went to school to become smile doctors, not bookkeepers and accountants, so we hire bookkeepers and accountants to handle the finances for us while we concentrate on delivering beautiful smiles and making a visit to the orthodontist the best part of each patient's day. The one thing I require from staff I employ is that they do everything they can to accommodate our patients and commit to prevent cost from ever interfering with the ability of a child who needs braces from getting to get them. This is part of the reason that our office accepts Medicaid payment. My spectacular staff shares this philosophy, allowing me to operate each day secure in the knowledge that they are making orthodontic care affordable to everyone.

The consequence of my distance from the financial aspects of the business is that I am not well versed on the various insurance plans, comparative pricing, payment plans, and so on. My staff handles all that with delicacy and empathy, which is all I ask. Occasionally I discover, after the fact, that we have had to write off payment for services rendered, but while delivering treatment, I don't want to know the status of payment, and as a result I almost never do.

AN ALMOST GUARANTEE

I do know, however, that our office, like most orthodontic offices, offers a variety of payment plans that make orthodontic treatment relatively affordable. For example, as I mentioned previously, if your insurance covers $1,500 of a $4,500 treatment, a family could pay something like $500 up front and $150 per month for the next seventeen months. That is much less than a car payment, for a much shorter period, and often means the family owes nothing during the last few months of treatment. Moreover, unlike a contractor doing renovations on your home or a physician caring for your broken leg or your diabetes, the price we propose for services is the price you pay and not a penny more, no matter how long it takes or what complications flare up. (There are some exceptions, but they prove the rule.) If you lose your aligners, we order new ones without an added charge. If your brace breaks, we fix it without an added charge. If your treatment takes months longer because you have not been compliant with the instructions, we continue providing service without an added charge.

Families that engage us for orthodontic care never have to worry about hidden charges, upselling, bait and switch, or any other shenanigans. We want people smiling when their treatment ends.

One of the things I love about orthodontic care is that it works just about 100 percent of the time. You probably have yourself, or know people who have, ailments on which they have spent hundreds or thousands of dollars to treat but that never significantly improved. Or the problem is ameliorated for a while and then flares back up. Consider back surgery, often considered the most temperamental of all surgeries for a chronic problem causing debilitating pain in millions of Americans. The failure rate for back-surgery patients is estimated to be as high as 50 percent, meaning that half the people who undergo this significant medical intervention, with its attendant cost, report little or no sustained relief.[13] (The cost of surgeries like spinal fusion and laminectomies is estimated at between $50,000 and $150,000, though few patients pay the full amount directly out of their own pockets.)

What is the failure rate for orthodontic care? It is something in the vicinity of zero.

What is the failure rate for orthodontic care? It is something in the vicinity of zero. When we speak of failure in orthodontics, we are generally referring to the bonding agent on a bracket failing to stick, requiring that the bracket be reapplied. If the issue is with a front tooth, we have a patient come in and attend to it right away. If the problem is with a back tooth, we wait until the next appointment. The

---

13   Anne F. Mannion and Achim Elfering, "Predictors of Surgical Outcome and Their Assessment," *European Spine Journal* 15, no. S93 (January 2006): https://doi.org/10.1007/s00586-005-1045-9.

entire operation of reapplying a bracket to a tooth takes a few minutes. That is the closest most orthodontists come to "failure." At the end of a patient's orthodontic experience, they have a beautiful smile and teeth that align for a perfect bite. They can chew and smile exactly as promised. Patients literally do look like the photo on the brochure.

It is not uncommon for patients to return to our office a decade or two after treatment, all grown up and deep into their career, still wearing the bonded retainer we installed at the conclusion of treatment. They come by to say hello, reminisce, and get some minor repair—at no charge, of course. Invariably, their smile looks great, and they are thankful to us. I can't think of a single instance in thirty years in which a former patient has returned to complain about their desultory results. You think a surgeon can say that? A car mechanic? A cable repairman?

Just recently I took my car in because it was not running right. The mechanic charged me a couple of hundred dollars to jingmajang the whimwham and sent me on my way. A few days later the problem reappeared, and after a few days' wait I was able to bring the car back. This time the mechanic adjusted the amalgamated clinger arm assembly and told me my left springer pylon coil was wearing out, charged me another couple of hundred bucks and said I should be good for the time being. When the issue persisted, I brought it back. This time, the mechanic agreed not to charge me for labor because the problem should have been fixed after two repairs, but he discovered that my condensifying compressure ramchain needed to be replaced, at a cost of four hundred bucks. When I got the car back, its performance was improved, not 100 percent; I am out $800 and have no doubt that sometime in the not-too-distant future a related problem will arise, and when I take it to a different mechanic, he will tell me that the whimwham should never have been jingmajanged and the ramchain that was replaced was not the issue.

Does the broad outline sound familiar, perhaps with different parts whose names are equally foreign to you? (I made up all those parts, in case you hadn't deduced that.) You have probably experienced something similar, laid out a pile of cash, and wondered what exactly that accomplished. No one ever feels that way at the orthodontist. When we promise a beautiful smile, a cure for your chewing problems, and realignment of your jaw for proper functioning, that is as close to always the result as life allows. When it comes to orthodontic care, you get exactly what you pay for—unless you get more.

So for a few bucks down and a small payment a month, we make people feel like Jennifer. I'll let her have the final words, and you can decide for yourself whether orthodontic treatment is worth the money.

"My husband always called me Miss America. When I got braces, I began to feel like Miss America. And when Clark took the braces off, I felt that I deserved to wear the crown."

TAKEAWAYS

→ The real cost of orthodontic care is significantly less than it was thirty or forty years ago even though the treatment is faster, more comfortable, and produces more precise and consistent results.

→ Dental insurance may now cover part of the cost of orthodontic care, something unheard of thirty years ago.

→ Orthodontic treatment is an investment in your child's future. We know that people perceived as physically attractive are more successful than those who are not.

➡ There is massive emotional pain caused to a person by the feeling that their smile diminishes their physical attractiveness. Research shows the lengths teen girls go to when they feel bad about their appearance.

➡ Most orthodontists have payment plans that take some of the sting out of the cost, and many are forgiving about families who need to postpone payments or pay less for a while.

➡ The price quoted for orthodontic treatment is the final amount. Patients do not discover halfway through treatment that they need more services than they had agreed to.

➡ The success rate of orthodontic care is essentially 100 percent. There is no question, as there very often is in other kinds of medical care, whether the final result will be positive.

CHAPTER 10

"HOW LONG DO I HAVE TO WEAR MY RETAINER?"

THE HUMAN BODY is a wonder, an ever-changing interweaving of intricately complex systems acting interdependently to create physical, psychological, spiritual, and intellectual experiences while continually reinventing itself. It is responsible for amazing feats like birthing new humans, painting the Guernica, imagining God, and proposing the theory of relativity. On a more prosaic level, it produces the structures of the mouth—bones, teeth, gums, tongue, palate, and more.

The forces that do all this remain in motion our whole lives, but not beyond, contrary to popular wisdom. (Sadly, the talk show host and comedian Johnny Carson did not have it quite right when he quipped, "For three days after death, hair and fingernails continue to grow, but phone calls taper off.") No matter how expertly an orthodontist moves, aligns, and repositions a patient's teeth during treatment, the forces responsible for the original position and orientation will resume exerting themselves after the removal of braces.

There is nothing unusual about this in any other aspect of life. It does not take long after a new house is built for the walls to shift and move out of plumb. Ask anyone who renovates older homes: there will hardly be a ninety-degree angle in the entire structure. That is not a reflection of bad construction but of the forces of wind, gravity, and shifting ground. In a way, it is a miracle that the world's great edifices continue to stand at all.

The movement of teeth after the completion of treatment is the very issue, you might recall, that Zia Chishti confronted, prompting him to invent Invisalign. It is the reason that orthodontic intervention does not end when braces are removed. There is one more step: wearing a retainer.

The purpose of the retainer is simple enough: maintain the progress made by braces for the rest of the patient's life. Over the past year or two with braces, teeth and sometimes jaws have been slowly coaxed to take up new residence in the mouth, but no matter how content they are in their beautiful new smile, there is always some part of them that wants to return home, even if that home was a dilapidated mess causing embarrassment and unhappiness. It is the mutable nature of our bodies.

Fixed retainers are, to simplify the process, a metal wire bonded to the back of teeth to hold them in place. With removable retainers, the wire is often in front of the teeth. In either case, their role is the opposite of braces—rather than move teeth to a desired location and alignment over a series of months, they prevent teeth from moving for the rest of life.

My own son Mitchell is the prototype of the noncompliant patient who fails to wear his retainer and discovers the consequences. Mitchell was a happy, vivacious, free-spirited child who listened only to the force of his own will. An artist at his core who played the violin and majored in vocal performance during his college years, Mitchell as a young teen was concerned with minimizing his time in braces and nothing more. At one point, although he needed more orthodontic treatment, he declared himself done, his smile good enough, and demanded his emancipation from the appliance. After resisting as long as I could, I finally capitulated and finished with the usual regimen: gluing a permanent retainer to his lower teeth and providing a removable retainer for the upper teeth, with instructions to wear it continuously for six weeks and at night thereafter for life.

I witnessed Mitchell's departure from my office into my wife's waiting car, but if that retainer remained in his mouth even the length of the car ride home, I would score that a victory for Dad. He never wore the removable retainer after that day, as far as I could tell. He was the ultimate cobbler's kid who had no shoes, but even if your father is an orthodontist, he is not a miracle worker and cannot force you to wear your retainer. You can see where this story is going, but Mitchell needed to experience it himself. A few years later he went away for a couple of years and returned with mild movement of the upper teeth that began to cause issues with his bite. Thankfully, he had matured a great deal by then, so in his twenties, he became his father's patient a second time and comported himself in a much more satisfactory manner. We completed the orthodontic treatment with clear aligners and he now wears his retainer, having seen firsthand the ramifications of not wearing it. In case you are wondering, there is no paternal satisfaction whatsoever in being able to point out to your progeny (but certainly not doing so) that you were right.

The general outline of this story plays out with an unfortunate regularity and leads me to repeat to my staff often that retention is the bane of my existence. While in my care, patients are to a large degree under my control in terms of their relationship with their appliances. Unless they are fully committed to flouting all the instructions of our kind and caring staff, patients are very likely to have a positive experience, and if they veer off the desired path, we still have the opportunity to gently guide them back. Once they leave, however, our influence over their behavior wanes, and the minuscule inconvenience of slipping an appliance into their mouth at night added to the microscopic amount of initiative required to do so may overwhelm their desire for permanent smile correction.

In short, patients who do not want to wear their retainer, even if they are the orthodontist's son, will not. The results may not be pretty.

In short, patients who do not want to wear their retainer, even if they are the orthodontist's son, will not. The results may not be pretty.

As a result, we aim to place bonded retainers in every patient's mouth. Because they are essentially permanent, unless removed by a dentist or orthodontist, patient initiative is not a factor. As they are taking up semipermanent residence in the mouth, bonded retainers work their magic every second of every day of every year of their functional life, preventing teeth from regressing toward their original position.

Unfortunately, not every patient is able to wear a retainer bonded into place. For example, patients with a tooth or teeth that have a short crown length or a deeper overbite cannot wear fixed retainers on the top teeth. This was the problem with my son, who was not interested in my desire to decrease the depth of his overbite with braces before graduating to the retainer.

Others decline the bonded retainer, primarily because it can complicate brushing and flossing. With the retainer sitting near the gum line, brushing and flossing require greater care and attention to cleaning the back of teeth. The appliance can trap food and bacteria, leading to the buildup of plaque unless the patient is diligent about brushing and flossing back there. Some patients, confident in their discipline to wear the retainer as directed, prefer to ease the chore of brushing and flossing. There is no difference in results with a removable retainer as long as the patient adheres to the regimen.

I should acknowledge here that this entire screenplay is based on nothing more than the hubris and paranoia of orthodontists. As I mentioned, things in life change. You don't see automobile dealers worrying about the depreciation of every car driven off their lot. Indeed, it is the very basis of their ongoing enterprise. When an ortho-pedist sets a child's broken arm, he does not guarantee it will never break again. Lasik surgery corrects people's vision—until it does not. As we age, we lose some visual acuity and close-up vision naturally, irrespective of the laser correction. Only orthodontists tear their hair out about the inevitable effects of change on their work. It makes no sense: even Michelangelo's Sistine Chapel frescoes require touch-up every few centuries. I acknowledge this, and yet I am so infected with the perfection bug that I lose sleep over the lack of compliance with our instructions to wear the retainer. (The option of pulling out hair has been foreclosed upon for years. See my photo on the book flap.)

SO, HOW LONG MUST I WEAR IT?

Patients regularly ask me how long they must wear their retainer, and I always proffer the same semifacetious answer: "How long do you want your teeth to remain straight?" It is generally true that teeth do not have a timetable; they move whenever the spirit strikes. Teeth do not achieve some magical point of no return when they become cemented into place, never again to shift. The mouth is constantly in motion, and absent a retainer, teeth are always inclined to exit the perfection that the orthodontist has created.

People often conceive of teeth as if they are posts positioned deep in the ground and secured for eternity with concrete. Once the concrete hardens, they imagine, the posts are permanently set in place, never to shift. This isn't wholly realistic even for posts bound in concrete, which do shift if some force is exerted upon them over sufficient time. In any case, this is not the proper metaphor for teeth of any mammal, which are held in place by a periodontal ligament that allows the tooth just a smidgen of wiggle room to withstand the rigors of everyday life. The superior analogy is a house built in an earthquake zone, where flexibility and ductility, rather than stiffness and solidity, are the keys to surviving seismic activity. Buildings that sway with the shaking of the ground are much more likely to endure than structures hardened against superior forces. Employing the same philosophy, teeth under constant forces inside the mouth have just a tad of "give" to them, allowing them to last the animal's lifetime.

The downside of this arrangement is that eventually, with enough back-and-forth force on the ligament, it weakens and allows more and more movement in the tooth, just as shaking a fence post does. A retainer helps hold the tooth in place against everyday stressors, as does a strong palatal arch. As any architect can testify, the semicircular structure distributes compression and dissipates tensional force outward, making the arch one of architecture's most stable and durable building forms. Conveniently, the upper part of our mouth comprises an arch, adding structural integrity to the supports for our teeth. Orthodontists attempt to strengthen that palatal arch by lengthening and widening it when necessary. Over the course of our lives, the arch tends to narrow and shorten unless a retainer is in place to prevent movement and maintain its stability.

Research by Dr. Robert Little at the University of Washington found that crowding in the mouth will naturally increase over time irrespective of the type of orthodontic procedures performed or other treatment variables. "The degree of postretention anterior crowding is both unpredictable and variable and no pretreatment variables either from clinical findings, casts, or cephalometric radiographs before or after treatment seem to be useful predictors," he reports in his research.[14] The upshot is, structures change, teeth shift unpredictably, and the only thing that positively prevents this is wearing a retainer religiously.

In fact, my own father, after removing my braces forty years ago, neither required me to wear a retainer nor bonded one into place. I never did think to ask him the reason for that decision, and now I am left to wonder whether he knew something that I don't know after all my years in the profession—or just got lucky. My teeth have shifted slightly over the decades but not enough to cause me either difficulty or a material degradation of my smile. Some people do get lucky, but wearing a retainer is insurance against that luck running out. As the play on the biblical verse goes, the race isn't always to the swift, nor the battle to the strong … but that's the way to bet.

Because retention is a key ingredient in orthodontics and the capstone on our service, we place a priority on getting it right. Although we make every effort to empower our adolescent patients, we make an exception when it comes to the retainer. We offer parents the choice of bonded or removable retainers for their children, and

---

14   Robert M. Little, "Stability and Relapse of Mandibular Anterior Alignment: University of Washington Studies," *Seminars in Orthodontics* 5, no. 3 (September 1999): 191–204, https://doi.org/10.1016/S1073-8746(99)80010-3.

on the basis of our recommendation, 99 percent choose the bonded retainers. They do not want to be placed in a position where they are constantly hounding their children to wear their retainer through their teen years. Adults are more varied in their choice, presumably because they trust themselves to wear the retainer.

I like to say that I have a policy on the matter: it is a policy of lifelong retention.

We are well aware that retainers probably have a statute of limitations in people's lives. A patient who gets braces at age twelve will very likely, at some point in their forties, fifties, or whatever, decide they are done with the retainer, whether bonded or removable. Retainers have a shelf life of maybe fifteen years amid the turbulence inside the biting, chewing, speaking, coughing, sneezing, spitting, swallowing, and raspberry-making machine that is the mouth. We periodically see patients a decade or two after treatment whose retainers have worn out. Following our lifetime retention policy, we repair them, usually free of charge. Even glued to the teeth, that appliance is taking a beating and will eventually give up the ghost. That is the one time a bonded retainer is "removable."

RETAINER MISCONCEPTIONS

After decades in the profession, I have heard most if not all of the misconceptions about shifting teeth postbraces. Remember that teeth are like new cars that depreciate as soon as you drive them off the lot. They begin to shift the moment the braces come off, and only faithful retention can positively prevent it. Nonetheless, I hear patients say that their teeth have shifted because their orthodontist removed their braces too soon. There is no minimum daily allowance of braces; they come off when teeth are completely corrected and the smile perfected.

More time in braces is never indicated after perfection is reached. The movement of teeth is natural and will occur unless retainers go in and stay in.

I have also heard people complain that the eruption of wisdom teeth has shifted their dental pattern and unraveled the work of the orthodontist. Although this complaint has more merit, because most humans lack the space for wisdom teeth to come in, their impact alone is not sufficient to undo the work of braces. Tooth movement is a multi-variable proposition dependent on many forces, most more powerful than the addition of wisdom teeth. None-theless, because most oral cavities of people of European descent, and many of Asian and African descent, are too crowded for those last molars to join

In our office we consider failing a learning experience and make a special effort to get better at our craft as a result of it.

the team, I generally recommend their extraction. "When in doubt, take them out," is my policy, though of course this is an individual-ized decision made collaboratively among a patient, their dentist, and their orthodontist on the basis of the specific crowding issues in their mouth.

In the early years of my career, I used a kind of retainer that featured a braided cable wire to hold teeth in place. It was the gold standard at the time, but over the years I discovered that the cable was not perfectly passive (i.e., it was pulling ever so slightly on the left canine). After removing the retainer and fixing that canine a few times, I abandoned that retainer and began employing a different kind. I have been using the new style for the last thirteen or so years and have yet to field a single complaint. In our office we consider failing a learning experience and make a special effort to get better at our craft as a result of it.

There is also now an Invisalign equivalent for removable retainers commonly called Essix after the company that makes the plastic. Made of molded plastic heated and vacu-formed over teeth, it is less cumbersome to wear than the old-style retainers. Orthodontists hope that Essix will increase the rate of retention and preserve those beautiful smiles that we have worked so hard to craft for our patients.

So here is the bottom line on retainers: Patients who do not wear them are going to experience some level of teeth reverting, perhaps not enough to matter but perhaps catastrophically so. In the worst-case scenario, the position and alignment of teeth will again become unacceptable aesthetically and functionally and will require a repeat of orthodontic treatment. We have treated a few such patients. One comes to mind whose noncompliance caused a relapse of crowding and misalignment in the mouth and resulted in the lateral incisor turning perpendicular to other teeth. Left alone, that tooth was going to wear a notch in the corresponding upper tooth and potentially lead to periodontic issues and the loss of teeth. We put them back in braces—fifteen years later—and installed bonded retainers so there would be no question about compliance or retention. We love our patients, but we prefer that they not come back for treatment a second time.

TAKEAWAYS

→ Teeth will begin to move the moment braces come off. Consequently, patients must wear retainers the rest of their lives.

→ Bonded retainers are glued into place and can be attached on top and bottom. They can complicate oral hygiene.

→ Not everyone is a candidate for bonded retainers on uppers and lowers. They may wear removable retainers that generally must be kept in continuously for a certain time, like six weeks, and then every night thereafter.

→ Teeth are always shifting, so retainers must be worn as long as patients want their teeth to remain straight.

→ Teeth move for a variety of reasons. Incoming wisdom teeth and premature removal of braces do not precipitate tooth movement.

→ There is now a clear plastic version, the retainer analog to Invisalign, that renders removable retainers even easier to use.

CONCLUSION

IT HAS BEEN my great honor and privilege over the last thirty-plus years to serve in the role I have alongside an extraordinary group of people. Every person who comes to see my crew and me has a need, whether simply cosmetic and ego fulfilling or necessary for ordinary life because they cannot bite or chew without our intervention. We are blessed to become part of our patients' lives and to make them feel more attractive, more confident, and generally better about themselves. We really do mean it when we say that we try to make the visit to the orthodontist the best part of our patients' day, but there is a corollary that we rarely talk about: our patients are the best part of *our* day.

Orthodontics is part science, part craft, and part art, but once a practitioner has mastered those elements, the greatest differentiator is the human part. We talk about best practices in our office daily, and we work hard to stay abreast of the latest techniques, procedures, and equipment. But the *best* best practice is kindness, caring, and empathy, and practicing that every day has made me not just a better orthodontist but a better husband, father, and person.

I hope this book has served as a guide to people—particularly parents—who are interested but skeptical about orthodontics. I have attempted to tell the truth and to be honest about my profession and even about my biases. My purpose in writing this was to create something useful for anyone who is considering orthodontic treatment for themselves or their children. I hope you have found it so.

ABOUT THE AUTHOR

BORN AND RAISED in Brigham City, Utah, Dr. Clark Andersen graduated from Box Elder High School. He served an LDS mission to La Paz, Bolivia, and speaks both Spanish and Aymara (an Indian dialect). Dr. Andersen graduated from the University of Utah with his bachelor's degree and went on to receive his doctorate in dental surgery cum laude from the Medical College of Virginia of the Virginia Commonwealth University. After completing a postdoctoral fellowship at Yale New Haven Hospital of the Yale University School of Medicine, he returned to the Medical College of Virginia to complete his orthodontic specialty residency.

Dr. Andersen loves living life to the fullest! When not straightening teeth, you might find him riding his road bike, raising money for local charities, running a marathon, cheering on the Utes, training CrossFit, sponsoring community events, coaching lacrosse, instructing scouts, riding his street surfer, reading to elementary school kids, or tearing up the slopes. More than anything, he loves hanging with his kids, grandchildren, and gorgeous wife, Susan.

CPSIA information can be obtained
at www.ICGtesting.com
Printed in the USA
JSHW042222130821
17852JS00007B/9